Praise for *Gluten Free Throughout the Year*

Gluten Free Throughout the Year *should be essential reading for anyone following a gluten-free diet. It's also an exceptional resource for people who want to improve their health, feel better, look more radiant, and learn how to truly transform their lives by changing the foods they eat. With its fresh ideas, elegant and nutrient-dense recipes, and creative, easy-to-follow tips, this book is a standout among many nutrition books on the market.*

- Nicole Brechka, Editor in Chief of *Better Nutrition* magazine

This is such an amazing book! It is just what the gluten-free community has been waiting for ... and urgently needs. Melissa gives us compelling evidence that we need a better gluten-free diet and then simply goes on to show us how to in masterful detail. It is a must-read for anyone adopting a gluten-free lifestyle. When you apply these insightful food strategies, you will indeed receive the "gift of gluten-free".

- Dr. Rodney Ford MD MB MS FRACP, Gastroenterologist, Pediatrician, Allergist, and Author of *The Gluten Syndrome*

Melissa Diane Smith has again produced a superlative resource for those who live the gluten-free lifestyle and want to achieve or maintain optimal health. She has served up a 24-month banquet of insightful recommendations for avoiding common miscues in this lifestyle.

- *Ron Hoggan, Ed. D., Author of* Dangerous Grains, The Iron Edge, *and* Cereal Killers *and editor of the* Journal of Gluten Sensitivity

Being gluten free is only one aspect of optimizing your health. Having a healthy diet is a much broader subject. Melissa Diane Smith will help you to fully understand both concepts. Everyone on a gluten free diet or who eats food should read this book.

- Dr. Stephen Wangen, Author of *Healthier Without Wheat* and founder of both the Center for Food Allergies and the Irritable Bowel Syndrome Treatment Center

Gluten Free Throughout the Year

A Two-Year, Month-to-Month Guide for Healthy Eating

Melissa Diane Smith

Copyright © 2010 Melissa Diane Smith

ISBN 978-1-60910-180-0

All rights reserved. No part of this publication may be reproduced, stored in a retrieval system, or transmitted in any form or by any means, electronic, mechanical, recording or otherwise, without the prior written permission of the author.

Book cover design by Todd Engel

Printed in the United States of America.

Against the Grain Nutrition
www.AgainstTheGrainNutrition.com
2010

Disclaimer

The information in this book is based on the author's personal experiences, professional experiences counseling clients, and opinions about eating gluten free and healthfully on a daily basis. The author is a health journalist and nutritionist, not a medical doctor.

The author and publisher are providing this book and its contents on an "as is" basis and make no representations or warranties of any kind with respect to this book or its contents. In addition, the statements made about products and services have not been evaluated by the U.S. Food and Drug Administration.

The purpose of this book is to provide general information for education and is not intended to be specific nutrition or medical advice for each person who reads it. The food products mentioned in this book are made with gluten-free ingredients. It's important to understand that some of the food products are made in dedicated gluten-free facilities and some are not. Some people who are extremely intolerant to trace amounts of gluten may react to foods that are not made in dedicated gluten-free facilities and therefore they should not eat foods that are not made in such facilities. Every effort has been made to be accurate, but food formulations may change without notice. For these reasons, always read food labels carefully, call specific companies when in doubt, and please consult with your own physician or healthcare specialist regarding the suggestions and recommendations made in this book and what is appropriate for you.

Neither the author or publisher nor any authors, contributors, or other representatives will be liable for damages arising out of or in connection with the use of this book. This is a comprehensive limitation of liability that applies to all damages of any kind.

It should be understood that this book is not intended as a substitute for consultation with a licensed healthcare practitioner, such as your physician. Before you begin any healthcare program, consult your physician or other licensed healthcare practitioner to ensure that you are in good health and that the examples contained in this book are appropriate for you and your particular health situation.

This book provides content related to physical and/or mental health issues. As such, use of this book implies your acceptance of this disclaimer.

*This book is dedicated to
gluten-free eaters everywhere,
especially those who are just beginning
to explore a gluten-free lifestyle.*

*A special dedication to my father, Don R. Smith,
an outstanding author in the sports arena, and
to my mother Helen G. Smith, a wonderful editor
and the person who taught me the most
about food and health.*

Acknowledgements

I am deeply grateful to Rodney Ford, M.D., Stephen Wangen, N.D., Alessio Fasano, M.D., Kenneth Fine, M.D., and Ron Hoggan, Ed.D., for their work in the field of gluten sensitivity and the enlightening interviews, talks or emails I have had with each of them – and to Loren Cordain, Ph.D., S. Boyd Eaton, M.D., Staffan Lindeberg, M.D., Ph.D., and other researchers who study the therapeutic value of grain-free diets whose work has also influenced my thinking.

Thanks also go to my clients and to the readers of my books who have taught me more about gluten sensitivity and the power of a healthy gluten-free diet than research studies ever could. And to Doug Levy, owner of Feast, for graciously sharing two delightful recipes for this book.

I also extend my gratitude to long-time friends and supporters of my work, especially Nicole Brechka, editor in chief of *Better Nutrition* magazine, Paul Teitelbaum of Programs Plus, who has consistently helped me through many technical issues, Jim Nelson for his invaluable photographic help, Margaret Cook, N.D., P.A., for her creative promotion of my work, and Kimberly Knost, who regularly shares gluten-free food ideas and news with me. And to the Southern Arizona Celiac Support Group staff and board of directors who have helped with much valuable information.

My heartfelt gratitude also goes to my entire family – Don, Ron, Rich, Marcia, Elena and Michaela and my uncle Bill – for their love and support. And a special thank-you to my cousin

Connie Caldes, a fellow author, for helping me with the publishing process, to my Greek grandfather Papou for handing down a love of tasty healthy food, and to my mother Helen for teaching me how to simplify recipes, for carefully reading and commenting on this manuscript, and for her steadfast belief in my work including this book idea.

Table of Contents

Introduction

Gluten-free eating is a growing movement. More and more people are realizing they can get far better results improving their health by adopting a diet that's free of gluten, a protein found in wheat, rye and barley, than by submitting to countless expensive medical tests and potentially harmful pharmaceutical drugs. That's big news for the United States whose general population is loaded with health problems. Eating gluten free helps overcome a wide range of medical maladies that even the best of modern medicine can't help.

An increasing number of consumers know this, even if their doctors don't. The number of people diagnosed with celiac disease, an autoimmune reaction in the small intestine to gluten, has increased in the past several years. But so has the number of people who do not have celiac disease but find that they have health complaints – everything from abdominal pain and bloating, to chronic fatigue, to migraine headaches – that are remedied by going gluten free.

The growing number of new gluten-free eaters has created more demand for gluten-free foods, leading to the gluten-free market growing at an average annual rate of 28 percent since 2004. Sales of gluten-free foods went from $300 million in 2003 to $1.3 billion in 2008, and market research publisher *Packaged Facts* projects double-digit growth in the gluten-free market through at least 2012. That means more new gluten-free foods and more existing food products that will be reformulated to be gluten free.

The Need for a Better Gluten-Free Diet

More new gluten-free foods means more choices and decisions about the foods you buy and how you put them together to create a gluten-free diet that promotes health. What you may not realize is that *for all the good that eating gluten free can do for people, it also can do plenty of harm if you eat gluten free the wrong way.* And plenty of people are doing just that. One study found that 82 percent of people gain weight after two years of eating gluten free, including 81 percent of people who were originally overweight. Many gluten-free foods aren't healthy, but many people who eat gluten free don't realize that because they are focused on gluten free and nothing else. To maintain health over the long term, it's important to be knowledgeable about other aspects of nutrition, too, and to know how to select healthy gluten-free foods and work them into your diet in all parts of your life – from eating in restaurants, to making a picnic, to what to eat and take when you have a cold or flu. This book will help you do that.

Through a diet guidelines chapter and a series of twenty-four short, easy-to-read articles, this book will teach you how to develop a more health-promoting gluten-free diet that you can maintain through all the months and seasons of the year. From my experience counseling clients, it takes time to learn all the do's and don'ts of a healthy gluten-free diet and how to personalize the gluten-free diet for you. These lessons are best learned on the job, in little snippets, as you follow a gluten-free lifestyle in real life. So, I have set up this book as a collection of month-to-month articles that will address common issues and questions that come up when most people start to eat gluten free – everything from other food sensitivities to how to get enough fiber on a gluten-free diet. Each short article will offer a personal story or brief introduction to a nutrition issue or a happening or event in our lives, followed by tips on how to put the information into practice.

Why Gluten Free is Becoming More Popular

Before the diet guidelines and month-to-month articles start, let me first fill you in on how and why so many people are going gluten free today. Awareness of gluten sensitivity by the public has spread like wildfire, thanks in large part to the Internet helping us share information and personal experiences much more easily. People who at one time never considered that they were gluten sensitive have gradually started to realize that gluten is a problem for them, too. The gluten-free lifestyle is a grassroots movement fueled mostly by the Internet, the great equalizer of the people – and it's spreading.

New research has also helped the growth of the gluten-free movement, showing what many people have long suspected: Non-celiac gluten sensitivity is a bona fide medical condition and the picture of celiac disease is much different than what was commonly thought ten years ago. People diagnosed with celiac disease today are more likely to have either no symptoms at all or symptoms formerly called "atypical" instead of the symptoms of diarrhea, weight loss, and malabsorption that most doctors look for. In adults, some of the more common presenting symptoms are constipation, acid-reflux-type conditions, bone disease, neurologic symptoms, and especially anemia and chronic fatigue. Children older than three who are diagnosed with celiac disease are more likely to have nongastrointestinal conditions, including type 1 diabetes, thyroid disease, Down syndrome, iron-deficiency anemia, short stature, or mood disorders. And it's more common to be normal weight or overweight than underweight when diagnosed with celiac disease.

But for every person who has celiac disease, there are seven to ten people with gluten sensitivity. Some researchers say the number of people with gluten sensitivity may be as high as two-thirds of the population. This is significant because people with gluten sensitivity experience uncomfortable symptoms just like people with celiac disease. In gluten sensitivity, the innate immune system, the most ancestral form of defense we have against "invaders," reacts to gluten, just like it does in celiac disease. In celiac disease, the adaptive immune system also reacts, but the adaptive immune system does not react in gluten sensitivity, according to recent research. Consider that the nervous system likely reacts adversely to gluten as well. Based on thirty years of experience working with patients and studying the growing research on gluten and the nervous system, Dr. Rodney Ford, a pediatrician, gastroenterologist and allergist from New Zealand, has concluded that gluten detrimentally affects the brain and nervous system that connects every cell and organ in the body and the damage done to the nerves leads to many symptoms in different parts of the body. While the exact specifics of how gluten provokes adverse symptoms are still being researched and debated, we don't have to wait to act on this information. Just know that gluten sensitivity is real, affects many more people than celiac disease does, and results in countless symptoms. The following, while not a complete list, is a list of some of the more common symptoms associated with gluten sensitivity.

Common Symptoms Associated with Gluten Sensitivity

Acid-reflux-type conditions
Anemia
Autoimmune diseases (including autoimmune thyroid
   disease, rheumatoid arthritis, and type 1 diabetes)
Depression
Bone disease (including osteopenia and osteoporosis)
Constipation and/or diarrhea
Fatigue and tiredness
Gas and bloating
Neurological conditions (including attention deficit
   hyperactivity disorder, headaches/migraines, and ataxia)
Skin conditions (including dermatitis herpetiformis,
   eczema and psoriasis)
Unexplained infertility

A rundown on diagnostic tests is covered in Appendix A, but the most important "test" you can do at this point is finding out whether your health improves when you eat gluten free. (Until more diagnostic tests become available, even Alessio Fasano, M.D., director of the Center for Celiac Research, agrees that this is an important way to determine gluten sensitivity.) If you have uncomfortable symptoms when you eat gluten, and they go away when you no longer eat gluten, you have discovered on your own (and inexpensively, I might add) that you are gluten sensitive and that the gluten-free diet is your best medicine. A gluten-free diet trial is much easier on your wallet than the expense of numerous doctor visits and diagnostic tests, and the treatment for gluten sensitivity – to continue not to eat gluten – is a lot less expensive than the pharmaceutical drugs people are prescribed for all of the above gluten-related symptoms and conditions. Therefore, if you have any type of unexplained illness that isn't getting better with medical treatment, it's a good idea to try a gluten-free diet and see if it helps you. [One caveat: This experiment works for virtually everyone except those who have silent celiac disease, a condition in which there is the damage to the gut seen in celiac disease, but these people experience few or no noticeable symptoms.]

Eating Gluten Free and Healthfully

If you're one of the growing number of people who find they experience better health by eating gluten free, then your only prescription is to go against the grain. When I say go against the grain, I mean of course to eat gluten free. But I also mean to buck the common mistake to eat gluten-free junk foods and too many sugars and gluten-free grains, and instead eat more vegetables, which are lower in carbohydrates and richer in nutrients than grains.

The next chapter outlines this and other diet guidelines to live by to improve your health and subsequent chapters show you practical ways to apply those guidelines in real life. Through school days, holidays, eating out in restaurants, traveling, and more, this book will guide you through how to eat smart with tips, recipes, and information you can use day in and day out to improve and maintain your health over the long term. Whether you read through this book quickly or just read one chapter every month, get started so you waste no time living gluten free healthfully throughout the year!

Five Diet Guidelines for Improved Health

People start eating gluten free to improve, protect, and even save their health. But all too often because of lack of information or poor advice from health professionals, they make nutritional mistakes with their diet that end up continuing their health problems or bringing them brand new ones.

It's best to learn how to do a gluten-free diet the right way when you first go gluten free. But many of us focus on avoiding gluten and nothing else, and then have to backtrack to learn healthy eating skills. Either way, this book will address issues that come up when eating a gluten-free diet and show you step by step how to eat gluten free for what it was meant for – promoting long-term good health – through different seasons and circumstances in our lives.

The following are gluten-free diet guidelines to live by day in and day out.

Guideline #1: Go gluten free naturally. It may be tempting to buy a lot of food products that are labeled gluten free, but the main foods you should purchase and have in your kitchen are unprocessed foods that are naturally gluten free, such as vegetables, fruits, poultry, fish, and lean meats. Stocking up on whole foods and learning simple ways to create meals with them are surefire ways to avoid gluten *and* to eat a diet rich in nutrients that supports health.

Guideline #2: Be choosey about the food products you buy. Gluten-free food products come in handy in our busy lives, but it's important to choose ones that don't sabotage your health. When selecting foods, look for those that are labeled gluten free and don't contain hidden sources of gluten, such as barley malt. (For a complete list, see the Unsafe Foods and Ingredients List at Celiac.com.) But also look for those that are made with little or no nutrient-poor white rice flour (often labeled as rice flour as opposed to brown rice flour) and starches, such as potato starch or tapioca starch. Even though these ingredients are mainstays in many gluten-free foods on the market today, regular eating of refined flours sets us up for nutrient deficiencies, unhealthy weight gain, and chronic diseases such as heart disease and type 2 diabetes.

Guideline #3: Become more unrefined. Besides refined flours, also try to steer clear of foods with other refined ingredients known to promote degenerative disease – namely, *refined sugars* and *refined fats*. Refined sugars include sugar (typically listed as "evaporated cane juice" on a food label), high-fructose corn syrup, fructose, and high amounts of natural sweeteners. Refined fats include vegetable oils (i.e., corn oil, soybean oil, cottonseed oil, safflower oil, and sunflower oil) and partially hydrogenated oil. To put this guideline into practice, seek out unsweetened foods as staples in your diet, and for special occasions, select gluten-free desserts that are sweetened with more nutritious sweeteners such as honey, maple syrup, or fruit juice concentrate, or with lower-glycemic sweeteners such as agave nectar or xylitol. Experiment with using better alternatives – fruit, stevia, or small amounts of mesquite meal, date sugar or coconut palm sugar – when making baked goods at home. With oils, completely steer clear of any food made with partially hydrogenated oil, limit snack foods and desserts that contain refined vegetable oils, especially corn, soybean and cottonseed oils, and seek out salad dressings and other foods made with olive oil.

Guideline #4: Personalize the diet for you. The gluten-free diet as it's typically prescribed is a good starting point, but it's not the end-all for most gluten-sensitive people. That's because it's quite common for gluten-sensitive people to be sensitive to other foods, too. You could have a true food allergy, in which adverse symptoms can develop within minutes – or have a delayed-onset food sensitivity, in which symptoms can occur several hours to up to two or three days after eating a food. Just like gluten sensitivity, allergies or sensitivities to other foods can cause a wide range of uncomfortable symptoms, such as gastrointestinal distress, nasal or sinus congestion, joint aches, or other complaints, and the only way to clear up the problem and improve health is to avoid the offending food. Some of the more common food allergies are to cow's milk, soy, peanuts, eggs, and yeast. Adapt the gluten-free diet to promote your best health by identifying and avoiding the particular foods that are problems for you.

Guideline #5: Eat more against the grain than you're used to. The Western diet that we have grown up on and are accustomed to is high in high-carbohydrate, wheat-based foods, such as bread, pasta, baked goods, and snack foods – foods that spike blood sugar levels and set us up for weight gain and insulin-related health conditions. When we go gluten free, most of us think all we have to do is replace the wheat-based foods we were eating with gluten-free versions of those foods. Gluten-free grains are free of gluten, but they are still high in carbohydrates. They also contain antinutrients that interfere with the absorption of key minerals and that disturb healthy digestive function when eaten in excess. By contrast, non-starchy vegetables – those that aren't root vegetables or hard winter squash – have four to forty times fewer carbohydrates than grains on a per-cup or per-serving basis, and they're much higher in vitamins and minerals. It goes against the type of diet most of us are used to, but it's important to fight the tendency to trade a standard Western high-grain diet for a gluten-free, high-grain diet. Instead, eat more vegetables in place of grains. That is the nutrition secret to long-term weight control and optimal health that most Americans, including those who eat gluten free, are missing.

Periodically remind yourself of these five guidelines. You'll see how they take practical form in the chapters that follow in the rest of the book. It takes time to apply the guidelines in everyday life and it takes persistence to keep applying them. The rest of the book will show you exactly how to do that.

Chapter 1 – January:

Heartier Breakfasts to Start Your Day

When it's cold outside, there is nothing quite as satisfying as warm, hearty food to start the day. Breakfast is our most important meal because it's our first meal after the longest stretch of time we've gone without food the whole day. Many people raised on an American diet think of sugar-sweetened cereal or baked goods as regular breakfast fare. But these foods spike our blood sugar levels, and the body responds by lowering blood sugar levels. Then we end up hungry or lacking energy just a few hours later. This happens whether the cereals or baked goods are made from wheat and other gluten grains or from common gluten-free grains such as corn and rice.

The key to replenish your body's energy, get your day off to a good start, and keep yourself going longer until lunchtime, especially during chilly weather, is to eat gluten-free foods that give you more staying power. Try these tips:

• **Think outside the box.** Train yourself to imagine breakfast beyond ready-to-eat cereal, baked goods made out of mixes of refined gluten-free flours (i.e., white rice flour, potato starch and tapioca starch) and high-carbohydrate gluten-free flours (i.e., brown rice flour, corn meal, millet flour, and sorghum flour), and rice-based hot cereal. All tend to prompt quick blood sugar highs followed by quick blood sugar lows. Instead, experiment with more nutritious grains and grain alternatives, such as quinoa, buckwheat, and teff, and get out of the habit of thinking hot cereal always has to be made sweet – with fruit and maple syrup, for example. The alternative grains often tend to taste better when they're made nutty (with nuts or nut butters added into them) or savory (with onions, shallots, tomatoes or gluten-free tamari sauce). Leftover cooked alternative grains also can be added to pancake batter to make heartier and more nutritious pancakes, especially when nuts or nut butters are also included – or use nut flour to make higher-protein, lower-carbohydrate pancakes for more sustained energy.

- **Power up with protein.** If a cooked cereal, no matter how nutritious, doesn't sustain you until lunch, then go for some protein, a slower-burning fuel, at breakfast. Poached eggs on either sautéed vegetables or a heartier gluten-free toast are traditional options, or have gluten-free turkey sausage patties served with fruit or sautéed vegetables on the side. For a dish with amazing variety, make a hash by cooking potatoes or cooked grain, assorted vegetables, and savory ingredients such as onions and herbs – with or without meat – in olive oil. You also can combine eggs, cooked grain, vegetables and herbs to make tasty patty-like croquettes.

- **Try dinner leftovers.** Break out of the mindset that breakfast can only be composed of traditional breakfast foods. Breakfast should be any food that gets you off to a good start. Once you wrap your mind around that concept, reheated dinner leftovers may work best for you. Whether dinner a night or two before was pork roast and green beans, a chicken stir-fry, or baked turkey breast with brown rice and vegetable pilaf, these meals make good breakfasts because they provide protein, fat and carbohydrates that are slower-burning than those in traditional breakfast cereal and toast. Plus, the dishes are quick and easy to reheat. During warmer months or when you're short on time, just grab a few slices of cooked chicken or pot roast, an apple or some celery sticks, and a few nuts. It's a different type of breakfast but a nutritious, balanced one nonetheless.

Here's a quick, versatile, easy-to-make breakfast recipe that's a great way to use up leftovers. You can vary its flavor by using different herbs, vegetables and/or meat. Try sautéing in chicken, turkey or pork meat pieces, or serve with gluten-free turkey sausage on the side or mixed into the hash for a festive Sunday brunch.

Savory Quinoa Hash

2 Tbsp. organic extra virgin olive oil
3 Tbsp. finely chopped yellow onion

1 cup cooked organic quinoa

3 Tbsp. finely chopped pecans

1/4 tsp. ground thyme

1/8 tsp. unrefined sea salt (I like Real Salt) or more
to taste

1-2 tsp. chopped fresh parsley

Heat olive oil in a skillet on medium. Add the chopped onions
and sauté for 30 seconds. Add the cooked quinoa, pecans and
thyme, spread mixture across pan, and cook without stirring for
45 seconds. Then stir mixture and sauté about 2 to 3 minutes
until golden brown. Take skillet off burner, mix salt into the
mixture, serve, and sprinkle with parsley. Serves 2.

---

*To gradually get the sugar out of your diet for improved health,
retrain yourself to appreciate baked goods with little or no
sweetening. There's no good reason to put concentrated
sweeteners in pancake batter, and most people top pancakes
with fruit, which is naturally sweet, anyway.*

*I adapted this recipe from a recipe for Almond Pancakes on the
back of a Dowd & Rogers California Almond Flour package. I
liked the recipe because it was simple, but with agave nectar in
the original recipe, I knew it would be entirely too sweet. I*

simply added unsweetened applesauce instead of agave nectar and a little less water and the pancakes come out with a similar texture to what many people are used to in pancakes and are still subtly sweet. If these pancakes don't taste sweet enough to you, give it a little time. Our taste for sweetness can change far more quickly and dramatically than you might imagine.

Almond Pancakes

2 eggs
1 tsp. gluten-free vanilla extract or vanilla flavor
1/2 cup unsweetened applesauce
1/4 cup water
1-1/2 cups Dowd & Rogers California Almond Flour
1/2 tsp. unrefined sea salt
1/2 tsp. baking soda

Beat eggs and mix in the other ingredients until batter is smooth. Stir almond flour, salt and baking soda into the batter. Oil a griddle or skillet with coconut oil over medium heat. Spoon the batter by heaping tablespoon onto the skillet. When bubbles on pancakes begin to open, flip pancakes over, and cook the other side. Gradually reduce heat on the griddle, oil griddle again as needed, and repeat cooking process with remaining batter. Makes 14 pancakes.

Chapter 2 – February:

Trouble with Dairy

If dairy foods bother you, that's not surprising. Cow's milk products are common problem foods for gluten-sensitive people for two different reasons: (1) lactose intolerance and (2) cow's milk allergy.

Lactose intolerance is a condition in which the body is deficient in lactase, the enzyme necessary to digest lactose milk sugar. It can develop because of the small intestine damage that occurs in celiac disease. When lactose isn't broken down, it passes into the large intestine, causing gas, diarrhea and other gastrointestinal symptoms. Once some celiacs remove gluten from their diet, the intestinal lining heals and they may produce lactase again and be able to eat milk products without suffering gastrointestinal symptoms.

However, one of the most frequent mistakes that people diagnosed with celiac disease or gluten intolerance make is assuming that a problem ingesting dairy products is due to lactose intolerance. "Unfortunately, a great many people who suffer problems when they ingest dairy products have an immune reaction to dairy and not an enzyme deficiency. This is a dairy allergy, not lactose intolerance," says Stephen Wangen, N.D., founder of the Irritable Bowel Syndrome Treatment Center in Seattle, Washington. If you have an allergy to cow's milk, eating dairy products – even if they are lactose-free or if you take a Lactaid digestive enzyme – will continue to cause health problems. The health problems may be digestive in nature or may be non-digestive, such as nasal congestion or earaches. The only way to relieve the symptoms is to avoid cow's milk products altogether. If you're one of the many people who experience better health by avoiding dairy, try these tips:

- **Be careful with the milk substitutes you use.** Some non-dairy beverages that are labeled gluten free, such as Rice Dream beverage, use a barley enzyme in processing and might contain minute residual amounts of gluten. Others, such as soy milk and Almond Breeze almond milk, contain soy, another common allergen. Many different non-dairy beverages contain evaporated cane juice, or sugar, which can provoke gas and digestive bloating in many people, especially people with yeast overgrowth, and should be avoided in general to protect against nutrient deficiencies, weakened immunity, weight gain, type 2 diabetes, and more. If you switch from milk to a commercial non-dairy beverage and still don't feel well, try eliminating the drink from your diet for a few weeks and see if your symptoms abate.

- **Try coconut milk or homemade nut milk.** Generally speaking, the milk alternatives with the fewest ingredients are the best tolerated. Lite or regular coconut milk works well as a milk or cream substitute in many recipes, for topping cereal or fruit, and for mixing into coffee or tea. If you're a bit more ambitious, make homemade nut milk with almonds or other nuts such as cashews or Brazil nuts.

- **Use olive oil, macadamia nut oil, or coconut butter.** Choose alternatives to butter that are appropriate for the dish. In Italian sautés and rice pasta dishes, organic extra virgin olive oil subs nicely. On fish and vegetables or in stir-fries, organic expeller-pressed macadamia nut oil is a flavorful, gourmet choice. And when baking, try coconut butter in place of butter.

- **Go for non-dairy frozen desserts.** For an occasional treat, choose from several gluten-free, dairy-free substitutes for ice cream, including Luna & Larry's Coconut Bliss and Turtle Mountain Purely Decadent Frozen Dessert made with coconut milk, and a few others that are available in some parts of the country, including Organic Nectars Raw Agave Gelato made out of cashew milk (OrganicNectars.com) and HeavenScent Almond, Rice & Agave Non-Dairy Frozen Dessert (GrowYourFamilyHealthy.com).

Want a sweet treat for Valentine's Day or another special occasion? Try this quick and easy-to-make rice pudding made with brown rice and no milk or eggs. I think the flavor gets even better after being refrigerated overnight.

Dairy-Free Brown Rice Pudding

1-1/2 cups organic coconut milk
3 Tbsp. honey
1 Tbsp. arrowroot powder
2 cups cooked organic short-grain brown rice
3 Tbsp. organic raisins
2 tsp. gluten-free vanilla extract or vanilla flavor
Ground cinnamon

Heat coconut milk and honey in a saucepan on medium until it starts to bubble. Whisk in arrowroot. Added cooked rice and raisins and simmer for 3 minutes, stirring constantly with a large spoon. Remove from heat and stir in vanilla. Spoon or pour mixture into small bowls or ramekins and sprinkle top of each bowl liberally with cinnamon. Cover bowls with covers or plastic wrap and refrigerate at least one hour before serving. Serves 4.

Chapter 3 – March:

Spring-Clean Your Diet

Spring is a breath of fresh air after the colder, darker days of winter. The snow melts, the days get warmer and brighter, and the flora and fauna of our planet bring forth new growth and new life. It's the perfect time to follow nature's example and breathe new life into your diet to regenerate your body and revitalize your health. Try these ways to give your gluten-free diet a thorough spring cleaning.

- **Pitch excess baggage in your diet.** If you haven't cut refined foods out of your diet yet, now is the perfect time to start anew by eliminating refined flours, sugars and fats – foods that weigh down the body with nutrient-poor calories and present numerous risks to health. Gluten-intolerant people naturally avoid one of the disease-promoting bad guys – white-flour (wheat) products – but there are others on the list: refined gluten-free flours, such as white rice flour; sugar and other sweeteners, such as high-fructose corn syrup; partially hydrogenated oils; and refined vegetable oils, such as soybean, corn and cottonseed oils. To shed unwanted pounds and help the body function at its tip-top best, wipe the slate clean on your diet and avoid foods with these processed ingredients.

- **Get in sync with the season.** Chinese medicine teaches that spring is the time to cleanse and rejuvenate the liver and improve the body's detoxification process. To do that, avoid heavy foods (i.e., red meat and cheese), eat less, and eat lighter. Relish foods of the season such as salmon, trout, young chicken, dill, chives, asparagus and strawberries. Eat artichokes and consider taking milk thistle extract – both of which have liver-protective properties. Take a load off the liver by avoiding alcohol – even gluten-free alcohol such as wine – a drug the liver has to detoxify.

• **Make it a very veggie time.** Include more green in your diet than brown or tan. Reduce the amount of gluten-free grains and breads you eat and eat more non-starchy vegetables, which have considerably fewer carbs and calories per serving. Fun seasonal foods to try are baby vegetables – those young, smaller versions of common vegetables – everything from green beans to zucchini to broccoli. Also include the traditional foods of spring – greens of all sorts, including mixed baby spring greens, baby spinach, dandelion greens, watercress, chervil, and sorrel. According to Judith Benn Hurley, author of *The Good Herb*, these greens are European herbalists' prescription for spring rejuvenation. Dress greens lightly with the simplest of dressings, extra virgin olive oil and lemon juice or unrefined apple cider vinegar.

• **Get fresh.** Emphasize foods that are as fresh as possible. When the weather is still cool outside, cook fresh foods – steam, bake, poach, simmer, sauté or broil them. As the weather gets warmer, add more raw foods, such as salad greens or raw veggie sticks, to your diet. Eating more raw foods promotes detoxification and renewal but too many uncooked foods can weaken digestion and trigger excessive cleansing reactions, according to *Healing with Whole Foods* by Paul Pitchford. So, don't add raw foods too quickly, especially if you feel cold, the weather is cold, or your digestion is weak. Other foods appropriate for spring cleaning are gluten-free sprouted foods, such as flax bars and flax crackers by Go Raw and Foods Alive, and sprouted seeds, such as Go Raw Sprouted Sunflower or Pumpkin Seeds and Kaia Foods Garlic & Sea Salt Sprouted Sunflower Seeds.

With baby spinach and dill, this is a simple, springtime meal in one dish.

Filet of Sole Florentine

4 cups baby spinach leaves

1 Tbsp. extra virgin olive oil

1 cup finely chopped onions

Grated nutmeg

1 lb. sole, flounder, or other mild-tasting fish fillets

1 tsp. olive oil

The fresh juice of 1 medium to large lemon

2 Tbsp. dill weed or Spice Hunter Deliciously Dill
seasoning (a combination of dill weed, onion flakes,
lemon peel & chives)

Wash the spinach well, then steam it for 3 minutes or until wilted. Place 1 tablespoon oil and onions in a frying pan. Sauté the onions until barely soft, then add the spinach, sprinkle with nutmeg and stir. Arrange the fish in a single layer over the spinach. Drizzle lightly with lemon juice and 1 teaspoon oil, and sprinkle with seasoning.

Cover the pan, cook on medium-low, and check after 5 to 7 minutes. (Scoop underneath the fish and spinach mixture once to make sure it isn't drying out or burning.) Fish is done when it's milky in color and flakes easily with a fork. Garnish with lemon slices on top, and sprinkle with extra lemon juice at the table, if desired. Serves 3 to 4.

* Recipe reprinted with permission from Syndrome X: The Complete Nutritional Program to Prevent and Reverse Insulin Resistance *(John Wiley & Sons, 2000) by Jack Challem, Burton Berkson and Melissa Diane Smith.*

Chapter 4 – April:

Having Problems with Corn?

When Kimberly Knost, a 53-year-old mother and office worker, began a gluten-free diet a year and a half ago, the gluten-induced acid reflux pain in her stomach went away. She began substituting corn products, the easy alternative to gluten-containing wheat products. But new problems emerged. "When I started eating corn tortillas, corn chips, popcorn or cornbread, it was hard for me to stop," Kimberly said. "I craved them, kept eating them, got very bloated in my abdomen, and gained weight."

After watching the documentary movie *King Corn*, Kimberly learned more. "I had no idea that corn is in practically every food in the U.S. food system and it's a big reason why Americans are so fat. After seeing that movie, I have tried to be very careful with my diet." Today, Kimberly mostly avoids corn to keep her eating habits and weight in control and buys more grass-fed meat. When she does eat corn, she goes out of her way to make sure it is not genetically modified and tries to have cut corn, which is less addictive to her than cornmeal or corn-flour products.

Kimberly is one of a growing number of gluten-free eaters who find that even though corn is gluten free, it cannot be eaten with abandon. Corn is a high-carbohydrate, high-glycemic (blood-sugar-spiking) food and eaten in excess it fattens us up just as it fattens up cattle. Two other issues: The production of commercial corn uses a lot of pesticide and the majority of corn in our food supply is now genetically engineered.

So, what kind of role should corn play in your diet? Use the following tips to educate yourself and decide the individual answer that is best for you.

• **Consider eliminating all corn products** for a few weeks to see how you feel, especially if you have gained weight or developed new health problems you didn't have before you increased your corn intake. During the first several days of a corn-elimination experiment, some people have strong cravings for corn-based foods, but cravings and other symptoms may lift, and weight loss often occurs, after four or five days. If this happens to you, you likely have an unrecognized corn sensitivity or carbohydrate sensitivity or insulin resistance and need to avoid corn for your best health. This is a common but largely unrecognized problem, especially in the United States where corn is unknowingly eaten so often.

• **Buy organic.** If you recognize no changes in symptoms or weight while avoiding corn, make sure you avoid the pesticides commonly used on corn and eat corn that is not genetically modified by seeking out corn products that are labeled "organic," "100% organic," or "made with organic ingredients" and that also specifically say "non-GMO."

• **Eat more blue corn or white corn**. Fortunately, these types of corn are not genetically engineered.

- **Put variety in your gluten-free diet.** Instead of eating yellow corn products over and over again, alternate various gluten-free products (i.e., quinoa, brown rice, heirloom rices by Lotus Foods, rice-based bread, and blue corn tortillas) in your diet. Also, try low-glycemic flax crackers or Beanitos bean-based chips in place of corn chips and especially use more vegetables, which are lower in carbohydrates, in place of corn products.

These muffins are lower in carbs and higher in fiber than most corn muffins and have just a touch of corn taste. With just three tablespoons of organic blue corn meal, this is a good recipe to try when reintroducing corn after an elimination trial. Serve with chicken soup or chili, or a large salad, or use as a side dish with baked pork chops or chicken breasts and steamed vegetables.

Light Blue Corn Muffins

3 large eggs
3 Tbsp. organic extra virgin coconut oil or
    organic butter, warmed to be a liquid
1 Tbsp. honey

2 Tbsp. apricot-applesauce or unsweetened
applesauce
1/2 tsp. gluten-free vanilla extract
1/4 tsp. unrefined sea salt
3 Tbsp. organic blue corn meal
2 Tbsp. organic coconut flour
1/4 tsp. Featherweight Baking Powder

Whisk together eggs, coconut oil, honey, applesauce, vanilla and salt. In a separate bowl, mix together the blue corn meal, coconut flour, and baking powder. Combine the dry ingredients into the liquid ingredients and mix until there are no lumps. Pour batter into greased muffin cups. Bake at 400 degrees for 10 to 11 minutes. Makes 6 muffins.

* Adapted from a recipe for Best Ever Corn Bread Muffins in Cooking with Coconut Flour *by Bruce Fife, N.D.*

Chapter 5 – May:

Breaking Out of a Vegetable Rut

Feel limited on your gluten-free diet? If you're like many Americans, that might be because you're eating a few familiar vegetables over and over again and don't consider all the other vegetable options you have to eat. Expand your thinking to broaden your diet. Start by trying these five vegetables that aren't commonly eaten.

• **Artichoke.** A member of the thistle family, which has tough petal-shaped leaves. Artichokes may seem intimidating to make and eat but doing so is worth it. Most people who try them love the flavor and the vegetable promotes health in many ways. Research shows that artichokes are rich in antioxidants and minerals and they help liver function, improve digestive disorders including indigestion and irritable bowel syndrome, and can lower blood cholesterol levels. To make them, use kitchen scissors to cut sharp tips off leaves if desired, cut off most of the stem, wash them in running water and drain. Steam them in a steamer basket inside a pot, making sure to add water to just below the steamer basket base. Steam until a fork inserted into the artichoke bottom goes in easily – about 25 to 45 minutes, depending on the size of the artichokes. To eat, pull off the petals and dip the white fleshy end in a lemon juice/olive oil/garlic/basil dressing, vinaigrette dressing, or gluten-free garlic mayonnaise. Pull the soft, pulpy bottom portion of the petal through your teeth and discard the rest of the petal. Continue until all the petals are removed. Use a knife to scrape out and remove the fuzzy part, then cut the bottom (the artichoke "heart") into pieces, dip, and eat.

• **Arugula**. An aromatic green with a peppery-mustardy to bitter flavor. Some consider it the star of salads and it is often served in Italian restaurants. Make a salad with it alone or add it to mixed greens. Dress with a balsamic vinegar/olive oil or lemon juice/olive oil dressing and, if desired, toss in Roma tomatoes, marinated artichoke hearts, fresh mozzarella or goat cheese, gluten-free pancetta ham, or glazed walnuts. Arugula also can be sautéed in olive oil and added to gluten-free pasta or can replace part of the fresh basil when making pesto sauce.

• **Bok Choy**. A type of cabbage with dark green leaves and white stalks that resemble celery. It's a natural to use in stir-fries. Slice the stalks like celery and the leaves into pieces. Stir-fry the pieces of stalk and other longer-cooking vegetables in macadamia nut oil for a few minutes, add minced garlic and ginger if desired, then add the dark green leaves for about 45 seconds, with salt or a few drops of toasted sesame oil or Bragg's Liquid Amino Acids, a gluten-free soy sauce substitute, at the end. If you're new to bok choy, start with baby bok choy, which is more tender and easier to work with.

• **Leek.** A member of the onion family that looks like an oversized scallion and has a delicate, milder taste. Cut them into 1/4-inch slices and simmer in soups, or sauté in olive oil or butter until they are soft but not brown. Cooked leeks can be pureed in a blender to make non-dairy "creamy" soups and sauces. They also go well in mashed potatoes or potato soup.

• **Spaghetti squash.** As the name suggests, this vegetable is good substitute for pasta and is considerably lower in carbohydrates and higher in nutrients. To prepare an average-size spaghetti squash, puncture with a fork several times and put on a baking sheet. Bake at 375 degrees. Turn the squash after 25 minutes and bake 20 minutes more or until the skin yields to gentle pressure. Allow to cool for 10 minutes. Cut the cooked squash in half lengthwise and remove the seeds and strings from the center with a spoon. Then use two forks to loosen the strands of squash, which look like spaghetti. Pile the "pasta" on plates and top with a homemade or gluten-free pasta sauce, or lightly sauté garlic in olive oil and sauté in the "pasta" and herbs. An average spaghetti squash makes 4 to 6 servings and you can freeze leftovers.

This recipe combines little-used leeks with more familiar vegetables for a delicious vegetable alternative to pasta. It's low in carbohydrates, rich in nutrients, and packed with flavor.

Vegetable "Spaghetti"

1 large carrot, peeled
1 medium zucchini or yellow summer squash
1 large leek
1/2 to 1 small green, red, yellow, or orange bell
   pepper (optional)
3-5 cloves garlic, slivered or minced
2 Tbsp. organic extra virgin olive oil
Unrefined sea salt and pepper to taste
Shredded fresh basil, chives, or parsley to taste
   (optional)
Prepared gluten-free pasta sauce (optional)
Cooked chicken strips (optional)

Cut vegetables into very thin (julienne) strips about 4 inches long. Heat oil in a large skillet or wok on medium-low heat and add carrots. Sauté for 4 to 5 minutes. Add remaining vegetables and sauté until vegetables are al dente, about 3 to 5 minutes. Season with salt and pepper, and top with fresh herbs and gluten-free pasta sauce and/or cooked chicken strips, if desired. Serves 2.

* Recipe reprinted with permission from Going Against the Grain *by Melissa Diane Smith (McGraw-Hill/Contemporary Books, 2002).*

Chapter 6 – June:

Taking a Vacation from Cooking

Summertime and the living is easy. At least it should be –
in the kitchen.

As days get longer, sunlight gets more intense, and
temperatures rise, it can get so sweltering hot that no one feels
like cooking. The good news is you shouldn't have to. It may be
nice to broil or grill some chicken kabobs, turkey burgers, or
fish on occasion, but you can get through most of the summer
eating nutritious, complete meals without heating up your
oven. Follow these tricks of the trade to give yourself a break
from cooking and make summer the coolest experience you've
had in years.

• **"Veg" out on salads.** The ultimate go-to, easy meal for
summertime is a big fresh salad. You can choose from a large
variety of greens (everything from arugula to spinach); salad
veggies (including cucumber, red onion, peppers, shredded
carrot, chopped celery, radishes, and artichoke hearts); and
other toppers (such as olives, toasted nuts or seeds, avocado
slices, or fresh fruit). To give your salad staying power, be sure
to include some protein, whether it's leftover chicken or fish,
chopped hard-boiled egg, beans, cheese, or gluten-free lunch
meats, such as Applegate Farms Roasted Turkey or Roast Beef.
Toss with a gluten-free salad dressing such as many in the
Annie's line – or make your own with extra virgin olive oil,

fresh or dried herbs, and either fresh lemon or lime juice, or vinegar (apple cider, balsamic, distilled, rice, or red or white wine). The varieties of salads you can make are almost endless. For a change of pace, make a no-fuss noodle salad by adding chopped vegetables and dressing to Sea Tangle Kelp Noodles.

- **Create sandwiches or wraps.** Start with two slices of toasted gluten-free bread, such as Food for Life China Black Rice or Bhutanese Red Rice Bread – or use just one slice for an open-faced sandwich. If you are carbohydrate sensitive or sensitive to all grains, make a sandwich with a Raw Makery Onion or Dill Rawtilla (a seed-based tortilla substitute), one of my favorite new products. Or forgo the bread altogether and make a lettuce wrap with a leaf of Romaine lettuce or Bibb lettuce as the wrapper. Add poultry or meat slices, thinly sliced tomato and red onion, and a dab of a gluten-free condiment of your choice, such as an Annie's gluten-free salad dressing.

- **Try other cool ideas.** Think outside the box of traditional cooked meals and prepare simple, fresh food. You can create homemade salsa or guacamole in about ten minutes with Melissa's Salsa Kit or Guacamole Kit (which contain all the fresh ingredients and recipe you need to create them!). Serve with cooked shrimp, gluten-free organic corn chips or flax crackers, and a variety of veggie sticks, such as carrot, celery and jicama sticks to make a light, summer-friendly meal. Or open a can of gluten-free fish, such as Wild Planet Low Mercury Wild Albacore Tuna or Sustainably Caught Wild Alaskan

Sockeye Salmon. Eat as is with lots of cucumber slices and some Kaia Foods Kale Chips for a super-quick lunch.

• **Savor seasonal fruit**, such as fresh cherries or nectarines. Packaged or canned meat or fish products give you cool convenience but they tend to be high in sodium. It's a good idea to emphasize potassium-rich fresh fruits and vegetables even more than usual.

Here's a refreshing dish to make when you are on your own and want something light and easy to fix. Serve as a side dish with a burger or a kabob and cucumber slices or celery sticks, or mix in cooked chicken pieces, tuna or salad shrimp.

Cool Noodle Tabouli for One

1/2 package Sea Tangle Kelp Noodles
2 green onions, sliced lengthwise, then chopped
3 Tbsp. chopped fresh mint leaves
2 Tbsp. chopped fresh parsley leaves
2 Tbsp. organic extra virgin olive oil
Juice of 1/2 medium lemon (or 1/4 to 1/2 more
    lemon as desired)

Unrefined sea salt to taste

1/8 tsp. gluten-free onion powder (optional)

2-3 large romaine lettuce leaves

Take noodles out of package and rinse with water. Drain and pat dry. Cut noodles into bite-size or smaller pieces. Add olive oil, fresh lemon juice, green onion, mint, and parsley. Mix well, then chill. Before serving, taste and add additional lemon juice and seasonings, if desired. Place romaine lettuce leaves on a plate and scoop noodle tabouli on top. Serves 1.

Chapter 7 – July:

Eating Out in Restaurants

When Colleen Kelly Beaman, niece of the legendary dancer Gene Kelly, was diagnosed with celiac disease 26 years ago, it was exceedingly difficult to get a gluten-free meal in a restaurant. Times have changed: Today Colleen has no problem speaking up and telling the restaurant staff what she needs. "The great thing is most people know what I'm talking about these days," she says. "It's definitely easier to get a gluten-free meal in a restaurant than it ever has been." Colleen is so comfortable and restaurant savvy now that she leads a lunch group once a month for her local celiac chapter and she eats out every day when she travels across the country and overseas to teach dance Kelly style.

To get safe meals in restaurants, you need to be armed with the right skills, knowledge and tools. Try the key strategies below to make ordering and receiving gluten-free meals in restaurants as simple as possible.

• **Scout out restaurants and their menus.** It's best not to go to an unfamiliar restaurant and not know what to expect. Plan ahead by first stopping by the restaurant and picking up a copy of its menu, viewing its menu online, or asking the restaurant to fax a copy. Read through the menu and look for dishes that have ingredients that are naturally gluten free (such as the Seared Halibut with Sautéed Leeks, Sundried Tomatoes and Tarragon recipe and the Fennel, Golden Raisin and Black Olive Salad recipe in this chapter). Also, jot down gluten-savvy questions that come to you, for example: Is this entrée made with flour? Can it be made without flour? What type of vegetable side dishes can I get instead of pasta? Then call the restaurant during off hours. Talk to the chef or manager, explain your dietary needs, and ask questions. Key restaurant personnel usually are very willing to discuss the menu with you as long as the restaurant isn't busy.

• **Consider getting a restaurant card to make communication with the chef easier.** Restaurant cards explain specific ingredients you can and cannot eat on your gluten-free diet. You give the dining card to your waiter and he or she will then pass the card on to the chef. Even a busy chef can look at the card and tell you which menu items are naturally gluten free or can be made gluten free. Several options of cards are available. A paper restaurant card is included with a paid membership into the Celiac Sprue Association (CSA). For a donation, printable restaurant cards are available from CeliacTravel.com. Sturdier, laminated, wallet-sized dining cards in ten different languages for ten different cuisines can be ordered from TriumphDining.com.

• **Go to a restaurant that offers a gluten-free menu**. Awareness of celiac disease has grown so rapidly in recent years that many restaurants now offer gluten-free menus. National chains that have this option include Outback Steakhouse,

Carrabba's Italian Grill, and PF Chang's. Regional chains include Bonefish Grill, Legal Sea Foods, Mitchell's Fish Market, Biaggi's Ristorante Italiano, Charlie Brown's Steakhouse, Claim Jumper, and Firebirds Rocky Mountain Grill. Some standalone local restaurants also are getting into the act. Do Internet searches or check with the Gluten-Free Restaurant Awareness Program (GlutenFreeRestaurants.org) or your local or regional CSA chapter to find restaurants that offer gluten-free menus in your area.

This is a recipe that the owner of a 29-year-old Greek restaurant that recently closed shared with me. It's a good example of a dish that's made with naturally gluten-free ingredients.

Seared Halibut with Sautéed Leeks, Sundried Tomatoes and Tarragon

8 oz. cut of fresh halibut filet

1-1/2 tsp. extra virgin olive oil

1 leek, julienne-cut

2-3 Tbsp. julienne-cut, sun-dried tomatoes

1/2 Tbsp. fresh tarragon

Splash of white wine (optional)
1 tsp. chopped garlic
1/2 lemon, squeezed
1-1/2 Tbsp. butter
Salt and pepper to taste

Sear halibut in olive oil in a sauté pan until golden brown on both sides. Place in a preheated oven at 350 degrees. In another sauté pan, place all remaining ingredients and sauté on medium-high for a few minutes until leeks become soft. Take halibut out of the oven when firm (after approximately 10 minutes), and place sautéed leek, sun-dried tomato and herb mixture on top of halibut. Serves 1.

Feast is a restaurant in Tucson, Arizona, that has a menu that changes every month and offers numerous gluten-free entrée and side dish choices and innovative vegetable dishes. Here is a recipe for one of those innovative vegetable dishes.

Fennel, Golden Raisin, and Black Olive Salad

3 heads fennel, sliced
Olive oil

Salt and pepper
1/4 cup golden raisins, plumped in boiling water
1/4 cup Kalamata olives, pitted and cut in half
1 Tbsp. lemon juice
1-1/2 tsp. honey
Chopped parsley
Fennel fronds

Toss fennel slices with olive oil and salt and pepper. Grill approximately 3 to 5 minutes per side. Spread out to cool. Remove core and cut into strips. Toss with raisins and olives and add lemon and honey. Taste. Correct seasoning and add parsley. Garnish with fennel fronds. Serves 6 to 8.

* Recipe printed courtesy of Feast restaurant, Tucson, AZ.

Chapter 8 – August:

Traveling Against the Grain

Ready to go on vacation? Whether you're going by plane, train or automobile, you can't just take off without thinking ahead. Traveling these days is stressful and often can be a complete nightmare if you aren't carrying your own food. That's even more true when you're gluten sensitive. (Just think of the airplane passengers who got stuck in an airplane on a runway without food for twelve hours!)

Keep in mind that getting to and from your destination is only half the challenge. To make your vacation days free from food worries and more enjoyable and relaxing, it pays to plan ahead and do a little research. Try these tips for traveling against the grain:

- **Bring food that sustains you.** This is an essential survival skill, especially when flying. Except on long domestic or international flights, airline carriers no longer offer special meals, and snacks that people can purchase in airport quick-food outlets, on planes, or along the road are all wheat-based. So, the only solution is BYOF – Bring Your Own Food. The most portable, sturdy, and nutritious snacks are nuts, especially almonds and Brazil nuts, which have a better protein-to-carbohydrate balance than most other nuts. Peanuts work well, too, if you aren't one of many who are allergic or sensitive to them. An apple, which is rich in blood-sugar-balancing fiber, is a good accompaniment. Also think of nut-based snacks, such as celery sticks with nut butter or a nut butter sandwich on gluten-free bread. If you're sensitive to nuts, try seeds, such as pumpkin seeds and sunflower seeds, and make snacks with unsweetened sunflower butter or hempseed butter.

- **Raise the bar.** Get to know the best bars out there and what they can do for you. Date-based fruit and nut bars, such as Larabar, Think Organic, or Nature's Path Dr. Weil bars, provide quick energy and serve as nice treats but are quite sweet and don't provide staying power. The original ReBar contains an impressive combination of vegetables and fruits in every bar, making it an antioxidant-rich snack to eat with nuts. Protein-rich bars made with brown rice protein, such as Pure Bar and especially Organic Food Bar (original or vegan variety), keep people going longer. They have been lifesavers on long trips for many of my clients. Mariel's Kitchen Blisscuits, which are made out of almond meal and coconut, also can be a stabilizing snack for some who can tolerate small amounts of milk ingredients on occasion.

- **Stay at a place with a refrigerator.** This is another survival skill that's especially important on long trips. The lodging you choose could be a hotel room with a mini-refrigerator, a suite or rented condominium with a full kitchen, or a friend's or relative's home. When you have a refrigerator that's handy, you can store gluten-free leftovers containing meat and vegetables from dinner the night before and eat them quickly in the morning before a long day of sightseeing, hiking, or whatever else you have planned. If you want to go further, visit a natural foods supermarket in the area, and purchase a few other handy refrigerated foods, such as gluten-free deli meats, prepared salads, and pre-cut carrot and celery sticks, to create outdoor picnics or mini-meals on the run during your vacation.

• **Research and plan ahead.** Just as you scout out restaurants in your hometown, you should do the same in the area you're planning to visit. *The Essential Gluten-Free Restaurant Guide* by Triumph Dining, with listings of restaurants by state and sample menus of restaurant chains that offer gluten-free menus, is a good place to start. But also do Internet searches for restaurants with gluten-free menus and for restaurant suggestions from celiac support groups in the area, and map the locations of restaurants and natural food stores. Print out the information and put it in your traveling bag so you have it handy on your trip. Good sites to check out include GlutenFreeTravelSite.com, CeliacTravel.com, Celiac.com, and Bob and Ruth's Gluten-Free Dining & Travel Club at BobandRuths.com. Investigating restaurants well before you go on your trip takes some time but it's worth it for giving you peace of mind, helping get you more excited about your trip, and allowing you to develop a game plan for working the restaurants you most want to visit into your schedule. Just like special attractions to see, special restaurants can make the difference between a trip and a real vacation.

If the more nutritious commercial food bars sold in health food stores are either overly sweetened or don't use the right ingredients for you, you can make your own food bar to take while traveling. Here is an idea for one type of food bar that has protein, healthy fats, vegetables and fruits, and is minimally sweetened. You can spread the batter on part of a cookie sheet and score it into bars, but I find the bars easier to make and handier to carry when I spread the batter into paper muffin cups. The bars soften and the orange zest flavor in them mellows the longer the bars are at room temperature in your purse or traveling bag.

"Carrot Cake" Power Bars

2 sample packs (4 heaping Tbsp.) Nutribiotic Plain
   Rice Protein Powder
4 Tbsp. Dowd & Rogers California Almond Flour
2 tsp. finely shredded organic unsweetened coconut
2 tsp. date sugar
1 tsp. ground cinnamon
4 Tbsp. Nutiva Organic Coconut Manna (a new
   creamy spread made out of whole coconut)
4 Tbsp. Nutiva Organic Extra Virgin Coconut Oil
2 Tbsp. organic unsweetened applesauce

2 Tbsp. shredded and finely chopped carrot
1 tsp. finely grated orange zest
3 tsp. organic raisins
2 tsp. chopped pecans or walnuts

Mix the first five ingredients together. In a separate bowl, mix the Coconut Manna, coconut oil, applesauce and orange zest, then mix in the carrots. Mix the dry and wet ingredients together, then mix in the raisins and pecans. Spoon and press the batter into six standard (2-1/2-inch) paper muffin cups, put the filled muffins cups in an airtight container, and refrigerate overnight or for a day or two. Put 2 mini-protein rounds each in three plastic bags before packing them in your purse or traveling bag.

Note: Date sugar is not really a sugar. It is made from ground, dehydrated dates. If you need a substitute, use stevia, xylitol, honey, agave nectar, or coconut palm sugar to taste. Also, if you have trouble making finely grated orange zest without getting the bitter white pith in it, invest in a microplane grater/zester, which helps make the grating process easy.

When gluten sensitivity specialist Dr. Rodney Ford and his wife Chris traveled to Tucson from New Zealand, we had dinner at

Feast and enjoyed a delicious spread of gluten-free food that included these appetizers, Quinoa Pancakes with Peanut Sauce. Feast chef Doug Levy graciously shared this recipe with me. The recipe calls for milk, but regular or lite coconut milk or another milk alternative can easily be substituted. I think the pancakes would taste good without the sauce as breakfast pancakes, too. If you aren't making a batch for a big gathering, half the recipe.

Quinoa Pancakes

3 cups quinoa
6 cups chicken or vegetable stock
1 Tbsp. minced garlic
Salt and pepper to taste
6 eggs
1 and 2/3 cups milk
1/2 tsp. salt
2 cups garbanzo flour
Olive oil

Bring the stock to a boil with the quinoa, garlic, salt and pepper. Simmer, loosely covered, until the quinoa is tender, about 35 minutes. Set aside. Blend the eggs, milk, salt and garbanzo flour in a blender until smooth, strain, and add to the cooked quinoa. Heat oil in a skillet over medium-high heat and spoon the quinoa batter into the pan to make pancakes about

2" to 2-1/2" in diameter. When they turn golden brown on the bottom, turn them with a spatula and cook to golden brown on the other side. Makes about 3 dozen pancakes.

Peanut Sauce

> 1/4 cup peanut butter
> 1/4 cup water
> 1/4 cup gluten-free tamari sauce
> 2 Tbsp. lime juice
> 2 cloves garlic, minced and crushed
> 2 Tbsp. rice vinegar

Combine all ingredients in a saucepan over low heat. (The mixture will become easy to combine as the peanut butter melts.) Continue stirring over low heat until ingredients are combined and mixture is smooth and creamy. Makes about 1 cup of sauce.

Serve the pancakes with peanut sauce with or without braised pork, and garnish with fresh cilantro.

* Recipes printed courtesy of Feast restaurant, Tucson, AZ.

Chapter 9 – September:

Gluten-Free School Days!

It's back to school time again – time to make the grade providing safe, enjoyable lunches and after-school snacks for your kids. It is a tall order to make food that is nutrient dense to maximize children's learning potential and food that your kids will actually like. It can be even more of a challenge to make food that is completely gluten free. Here's a little cheat sheet to help you!

For the Lunch Bag

• **Make sandwiches or roll-ups.** Use gluten-free bread to make nut butter sandwiches with apple or banana slices, fruit spread, or apple butter. Or try organic corn tortillas as the "bread" in roll-up sandwiches with gluten-free deli turkey meat, pizza sauce and mozzarella, chicken salad or any other filling your child likes. Be sure to include an ice pack if the filling needs to stay cold.

• **Pack dinner leftovers in a Thermos**. Warm meals that work nicely for kids' school lunches include homemade soups, brown rice pasta and meat sauce, Spanish rice, and stir-fries.

• **Include fun food**. Kids gravitate to food they can eat with their hands (i.e., Go Raw Sprouted Sunflower Seeds) or food they can dip into sauces (i.e., fresh veggie sticks with hummus or a gluten-free Annie's salad dressing, celery sticks with nut butter, or rice chips, corn chips or Beanitos bean chips with salsa). They also love sweets, of course, but opt for treats that are made without refined sugar and are more nutritious than standard fare, such as Go Raw Chocolate Super Cookies or Fabe's Organic Mini-Macaroons.

• **Get fruity.** The most nutritious, natural sweets are fruit. Include an apple, banana or orange in a lunch bag – or a homemade fruit salad in a container in a lunchbox. If you run out of fresh fruit, another good option is Kettle Valley All Natural Organic Fruit Snacks.

For Field Trips

• **Buy nutritious food bars.** Stock up on gluten-free food bars that are convenient for your child to carry on field trips, in the lunch bag and for after-school activities. One good choice is a fruit-based bar, such as a Larabar – a sweet, satisfying treat that is a good source of fiber. When your child needs a mini-meal to raise sagging energy levels, a better choice is a protein bar, such as Chocolate Chip or Cinnamon Raisin Organic Food Bar made with organic brown rice protein, or almond-butter-based Omega-3 Flax Organic Food Bar.

For After School

• **Teach your kids to get unrefined.** Gluten-sensitive kids, like most Americans, eat a lot of refined sugar and refined flour products – foods that promote sugar cravings, overeating, weight gain and more serious insulin-related health conditions over time. Break that trend by having nutritious whole foods around the house to munch on. Good after-school snacks include: grapes and toasted pecans; apple slices or Crunchmaster Original Multi-Seed Crackers with nut or seed butter; a mozzarella cheese stick and carrot sticks with salad dressing; an Organic Garden Herb Sunshine Burger (made with brown rice, sunflower seeds and carrots); or a hard-boiled omega-3-enriched egg and a bowl of blueberries topped with coconut milk.

• **Serve sugar-free beverages.** The easiest way to help your kids stay healthy, have steadier moods, mental focus, and energy levels, and not overeat or gain weight is to cut sugary drinks out of their diet. Try stevia-sweetened, low-calorie Olade, a beverage that comes in a variety of flavors and was developed by a man who has diabetes. Even better, serve more calorie-free water and sparkling mineral water with fruit essence.

Here's an all-in-one meal that is made more nutritious by using vegetable juice – and your kids will never know it or care! It makes great leftovers, too.

Easy Spanish Rice with Meat

1 cup long-grain or short-grain brown rice
2 cups gluten-free chicken broth
3 Tbsp. organic extra virgin olive oil
1 lb. ground dark-meat turkey
1/2 medium onion, chopped
2 garlic cloves, minced
1/2 green or red bell pepper, chopped (optional)
1-1/2 cups V8 vegetable juice
2 tsp. oregano leaves
1/4-1/2 tsp. Tabasco red pepper sauce (optional)
Black pepper to taste
1/3 to 1/2 cup organic Colby and/or Monterey Jack
   cheese, shredded (optional)
1 Tbsp. fresh minced parsley leaves (optional)

Cook brown rice in chicken broth (or make brown rice a day ahead of time and refrigerate). In a sauté pan, cook ground turkey and vegetables in olive oil until meat is browned and vegetables are tender. Add in the cooked brown rice, vegetable juice and seasonings. Raise heat until it starts to bubble, then reduce heat and simmer for 10 minutes, stirring occasionally.

Taste and add more oregano or Tabasco sauce if needed. Remove from heat and sprinkle with parsley and cheese if using. Serves 4 to 6.

Chapter 10 – October:

Jazzing Up Rice

Bored with eating plain brown rice? That's actually a common problem for gluten-free eaters. The monotony may seem necessary to eat safe foods, but fortunately, gluten-free life doesn't have to be so boring. There's a whole world of gluten-free rice out there and many different ways to make rice to change its flavor. Try these tips to shake things up, explore new horizons, and treat your taste buds to new tastes and variety:

• **Simmer in flavor.** Use a gluten-free broth such as Shelton's Organic Chicken Broth or Pacific Foods Organic Free-Range Chicken Broth or Vegetable Broth to cook rice in instead of water. Simmering rice in broth is an easy way to make rice pilaf without extra work.

• **"Veg" out and go nuts**. Sauté assorted vegetables or nuts in olive oil, butter or macadamia nut oil and add into cooked rice. Mushrooms and shallots; celery, onions and slivered almonds; spinach, garlic, sliced artichoke hearts and pine nuts – the combinations you can create are endless.

• **Sauce it up**. For completely different tastes, top rice with, or mix in, gluten-free pasta sauce, pesto sauce, wheat-free tamari or a coconut curry sauce.

• **Explore the world of rice.** There is a lot more than the familiar basmati rice and brown rice. Dive into trying each of these different types of whole-grain rice with their own special taste:

Bhutanese red rice – Grown in the Kingdom of Bhutan in the eastern Himalayas, this rice from Lotus Foods has a mild, nutty/earthy, slightly sweet flavor. It is semi-milled, meaning some of the reddish pigment in the bran that is formed by minerals in the soil is left on the rice. It cooks in just 20 minutes.

Forbidden Black Rice – The trademarked name for medium-grain Chinese black rice that was once grown exclusively for the Emperors of China. It is rich in iron and has a fragrant aroma, nutty taste, and dramatic black to deep purple color. Now available in certified organic from Lotus Foods. It cooks in 30 minutes.

Kalijira Rice – Grown in Bangladesh, brown kalijira is a tiny aromatic brown rice with a low glycemic index, meaning it provokes a lower blood sugar response than some other types of rice. It is a top-selling rice sold by Lotus Foods. It cooks in 25 minutes.

Jasmine Rice – An aromatic long-grain organic rice originally from Thailand but now also grown in the United States and sold by Lotus Foods and Lundberg Family Farms. It contains 10 percent rice bran that gives the rice a light tan color and it has an aroma and flavor that is similar to popcorn or roasted nuts. It cooks in 45 minutes.

Wehani Rice – Developed by Lundberg Farms, this fragrant rice is a reddish-brown hybrid of Indian basmati and long-grain brown rice. It cooks in 45 minutes.

Black Japonica Rice – An aromatic blend of Japanese short-grain black rice and medium-grain mahogany rice developed by Lundberg Family Farms. It cooks in 45 minutes.

Wild rice – The seed of a long-grain marsh grass that grows wild in isolated lake and river beds primarily in North America and also in similar regions in some parts of Asia. Lower in calories and carbohydrates than most other rices, it has a distinctive nutty flavor and chewy texture and is often used with other types of rice or other ingredients in rich and hearty gourmet dishes. It cooks in 45 to 50 minutes.

This dish works well when made with long-grain or short-grain brown rice but it tastes equally delicious when made with brown kalijira rice. It's perfect to serve with fish, shrimp, chicken, or lamb. If you're just getting used to more vegetables in your diet, you can start out using less spinach and gradually add more.

Greek Spinach and Rice

1 cup brown kalijira rice
1-3/4 cups gluten-free chicken broth
2 Tbsp. organic extra virgin olive oil
1 small yellow onion, chopped
4 to 5 cups of baby spinach leaves (stems
    removed, if desired)
Juice of 1 lemon
Unrefined sea salt and pepper to taste

Put the rice and chicken broth in a pan, turn heat to high until it starts to boil, then reduce heat to low, cover, and cook the rice until done, about 25 minutes. Add olive oil to a wok or deep-set frying pan, heat on medium, and sauté onions until soft, about 2 to 3 minutes. Add spinach leaves and quickly turn to lightly cook. (Spinach will cook down considerably from what it looks like when first added.) Add onion and spinach mixture into cooked rice with lemon juice and mix well. Add salt and pepper to taste and squirt with extra lemon juice if desired. Makes eight 1/2-cup servings.

Chapter 11 – November:

Celebrating Autumn's Bounty

This time of year there is much to celebrate and be thankful for – family, friends, and the flavorful, seasonal foods of autumn.

It's not helpful to dwell on the gluten-containing foods you used to eat on Thanksgiving. Instead, appreciate all the fresh foods you *can* eat. Use your need for a gluten-free diet as a golden opportunity to explore the naturally gluten-free foods of fall in all their abundance. Meals, side dishes and desserts that are made with seasonal foods have more color, texture, and taste than the bland white-flour products that end up on many Americans' Thanksgiving tables. As an added bonus, they have many more nutrients to keep you healthy.

Try these tips to experience the best of autumn:

• **Get back to some roots.** The traditional vegetables of fall are root vegetables that grow in the ground, including onions, garlic, carrots, parsnips, daikon radish, potatoes, turnips, rutabagas, sweet potatoes and yams. These vegetables store up energy and nutrients for winter and help us do that, too, when we eat them. As the weather gets colder, it's a good idea to incorporate more of these vegetables into your diet. Make soups or stews with small amounts of assorted root vegetables and get in the habit of baking sweet potatoes or yams to serve as side dishes with roasted meat or poultry.

- **Squash up your diet.** Another vegetable of fall is winter squash – a colorful food family that includes acorn squash, butternut squash, and spaghetti squash. You can bake squash whole or cut it in half first before baking. Or you can cut it into chunks and steam it. When the squash is done, top it with butter, flaxseed oil, hazelnut oil, or almond butter, and a dash of cinnamon or a tiny drizzle of 100% pure maple syrup. You also can fill any baked winter squash with your favorite gluten-free stuffing. If you want to bake or steam pumpkin – another member of the squash family – use the small, pie variety, not the large jack-o-lantern kind.

- **Explore the world of nuts.** 'Tis the season for nuts, so get creative with different types and ways to use them. The simplest way is to serve nuts in their shell with nutcrackers to crack them open – something that is easy for you, but festive and fun for guests. Other suggestions: Toast nuts in the oven to make easy, melt-in-your-mouth snacks or tasty toppers for salads, cereal, or baked sweet potatoes, yams or winter squash. Put chopped nuts into stuffings. Or make a special seasonal stuffing with chestnuts.

- **Highlight fall fruit.** Use seasonal fruit – cranberries, apples or pears – in special ways to turn ordinary salads, side dishes and desserts into festive foods of the season. Make cranberry sauce or cranberry relish from scratch. Add dried cranberries or sliced apple or pear to salads to give them extra holiday sparkle. Include chopped apple in stuffings, or make apple or pear crisp, crumble or pie with gluten-free flour. You and your guests will never miss the gluten!

Look for recipes you can adapt to be simpler. This recipe started as a recipe on a package of Trader Joe's butternut squash cubes that included blending the sauce at the end and adding cheese. I eliminated the blending and the cheese, added a bit more olive oil and seasoning, and cooked it a bit longer, and I was delightfully pleased with how it turned out.

Butternut Squash with Fresh Sage

2 Tbsp. organic extra virgin olive oil

1-2 small shallots, minced

4 cups cubed butternut squash cubes (or two 8-oz.
  Trader Joe's packages)

2 pinches ground nutmeg

1 bay leaf (optional)

6-8 fresh sage leaves, cut lengthwise into thin strips

2/3 cup gluten-free chicken broth

Unrefined sea salt and pepper to taste

Place the olive oil and shallots in a deep skillet over medium heat until the shallots begin to color. Add butternut squash cubes and season with salt and pepper. Sauté a few minutes until coated in olive oil and slightly caramelized on all sides. Add the nutmeg, bay leaf, fresh sage strips and chicken broth. Cover the pan and cook until the squash is tender but still holding its shape (about 8 minutes). If extra broth remains, cook down while stirring the squash or, if squash isn't done to your liking, remove dish from heat, leave covered, and allow it to steam in dish for a few minutes. Serves 6 to 8.

Want something easy to fix for your Thanksgiving meal dessert? Try this: personalized "sundaes" that people can make right at the table on Thanksgiving day! It's ultra simple and a big hit with guests.

Just start with sliced, perfectly ripe, fragrant and juicy Barlett pears and locally grown, shelled pecan halves that you home-toast in the oven. Have ground cinnamon, 100% pure maple syrup, coconut milk, and gluten-free, dairy-free frozen dessert at the table and let people choose what they want to add, customizing their dessert based on their own preferences and tolerances. That's it! Bursting with the unique flavors of fall, this is a great dessert to serve when you have guests that have many different dietary needs.

Pecan-Pear Autumn Sundaes

8 Tbsp. pecan halves
2 medium, ripe, organic Bartlett pears with the
  skins on
Organic coconut milk
Purely Decadent Vanilla Bean Non-Dairy Frozen
  Dessert made with Coconut Milk, or other
  gluten-free vanilla-flavored non-dairy frozen dessert
  or ice cream
100% pure maple syrup
Ground cinnamon

Preheat oven to 325 degrees. Put pecan halves on a cookie sheet, place the sheet on a medium rack in the oven, and toast the pecans for 6 to 9 minutes until fragrant and browned, being careful not to burn them. While the pecans are toasting, wash pears and cut off any bruised spots. Keep the skin on, slice each pear in half, and cut each half into very thin slices. Scoop out 1/3-cup frozen dessert for the guests that want it and place into bowls. In each bowl, arrange the thin pear slices from half a pear to the side of and on top of the frozen dessert, then top with 2 Tbsp. of toasted pecan halves. Place maple syrup and ground cinnamon on the table and allow dinner guests to eat dessert as is or add a few drops of maple syrup or a sprinkle of ground cinnamon as desired to create their own personalized sundaes. Serves 4.

* Recipes reprinted from Healthier Holidays Going Against the Grain *E-book by Melissa Diane Smith.*

Chapter 12 – December:

How to Have a Healthier Holiday Season

For all the happiness the holiday season can bring, it can present challenges to health, too. It's common to rush around, become anxious, forget to eat then overeat, come down with the latest bug, gain weight that you can't lose in the new year, and spend so much time in the kitchen that you miss out on socializing with people who are dear to you. The worst holiday downer of all – something unique to those of us who are gluten sensitive – is unknowingly eating a food that contains gluten, then getting sick and feeling horrible.

The good news is you can prevent all these common challenges and enjoy the healthiest of holidays. It just takes adjusting your attitude and actions to go against the grain, both figuratively and literally. Try these tips to follow the road less traveled to better wellness during this festive time of year.

• **Stock up on gluten-free staples.** Early in the season, buy extra amounts of the most important food products to you – foods you use often and can't do without if unexpected events prevent you from buying more. By planning ahead and loading up on staples, you won't have to scramble for ingredients at the last minute or get stressed if the product is out of stock later on. You'll also have grab-and-go snacks to quickly pack for traveling or holiday shopping at the spur of the moment. Common "essentials" are: assorted nuts and trail mixes; gluten-free food bars, such as Organic Food Bar or Pure Food Bar; gluten-free broth; and gluten-free bread or grains, such as brown rice, Lotus Foods' heirloom rices, or quinoa.

• **Stop the sugar blues.** Indulging in sugar-laden baked goods, candy and drinks, even gluten-free ones, can set you up for not feeling well. That's because blood-sugar spikes, followed by blood-sugar drops, can lead to tiredness, irritability, sugar cravings, and weight gain. What's more, eating sugar suppresses the immune system, leaving people more susceptible to developing colds, flus, and infections. Sure, sugary candy, baked goods and drinks abound during the holidays, but the less you partake of them, the better it is for your immune system and your ability to fight off illness. To enjoy some sweetness of the season without bitter health consequences, steer clear of nutrient-poor candy and sweetened drinks (i.e., soft drinks, hot chocolate, coffee or tea with sugar); have a gluten-free dessert only every so often, or split it with a friend after a well-balanced meal; reduce the amount of sweetener in desserts that you make; and include sources of blood-sugar-balancing fiber, such as nuts.

• **Keep meals as simple and easy as possible.** You can make stuffing by cooking up brown rice or quinoa, or drying gluten-free bread cubes in the oven first, then adding other ingredients and cooking some more. However, a little-known secret to reducing the time and work involved in cooking gluten-free is to eliminate the grain all together! Make a grain-free stuffing or an assortment of sautéed or roasted vegetables. Skip making a gluten-free crust ahead of time and prepare a pumpkin pie without a crust. Ditching the grains is thinking outside the box of what most gluten-sensitive people do, but it reduces steps in cooking and makes food preparation easier and less stressful. Also, prepare gluten-free foods that can be reheated or those that are served cold a day or two ahead. That gives you more time to join the party and enjoy yourself!

Part of the fun of the holidays is using small amounts of festive, seasonal foods in special holiday meals. Here's an easy recipe for stuffing that uses chestnuts – and peeled raw chestnuts are the key to the easiness of the recipe. The most convenient product is a jar of peeled whole chestnuts from France by Ardeche-marrons; it's found every holiday season at Cost Plus World Market. You also may be able to find jars of peeled chestnuts and frozen peeled chestnuts in other stores.

Chestnut Stuffing

1-1/4 cups peeled whole raw chestnuts
2-3 pearl onions, peeled and cut in half (or 4-5
   baby pearl onions, peeled)

3 shallots, peeled and cut in half

1 small or 1/2 large fennel bulb, cut in half, then cut
lengthwise into 1/4-inch-wide sections

1/4 cup organic extra virgin olive oil (or organic butter)

1 cup gluten-free chicken broth

1/2 cup fresh shelled walnut pieces

Pinch of rubbed sage (optional)

Unrefined sea salt and pepper to taste, if desired

Heat the oil (or butter) in a deep sauté pan. Add the onions, shallots, and fennel and brown slightly for a few minutes. Add the chestnuts, arranging them alternatively with the onions, shallots, and fennel. Add the chicken stock, bring it to a boil, then reduce heat to low and cover the pan. Let the ingredients simmer for about 40 minutes, stirring as little as possible so as not to damage the chestnuts. Remove the lid. Taste. Season with salt, pepper and sage, if desired. If there's extra liquid, reduce the liquid slightly (but leave some), then roll the chestnuts, onions, shallots, and fennel in the liquid so that they are covered in a shiny coat. (If extra liquid is needed, add a few extra tablespoons of chicken broth.) Cut any fennel, pearl onion or shallot pieces that seem too large. Add the walnuts, cover, and continue to cook the mixture, stirring every so often, for another 5-10 minutes until walnuts are softer, no longer have such a strong walnut taste, and have picked up the other flavors. Serve the chestnut stuffing in its au jus as a side dish for meat and poultry.

Feel like having stuffing but can't track down peeled raw chestnuts? No problem. Just make this recipe instead. The flavors of assorted vegetables meld to create this hearty, moist and savory stuffing that is perfect to make a day before entertaining and reheat the next day. It's also a safe side dish to bring to any potluck or holiday gathering away from home. The stuffing goes well with roast turkey, chicken, beef, or pork.

Savory Stuffing

5 pearl onions, peeled and cut in half
4 small shallots, peeled and cut in half
1 large fennel bulb (white part only), cut in half,
    then cut lengthwise into 1/4-inch-wide sections
1 celery stalk, cut lengthwise and chopped
    (optional; makes a lighter stuffing)
1/4 cup organic extra virgin olive oil
1-1/4 cups gluten-free chicken broth
1/2 tsp. rubbed sage
1/2 cup chopped walnuts
8-ounce carton of button mushrooms, quartered
Unrefined sea salt and black pepper to taste
1 Tbsp. chopped fresh parsley leaves
1 Tbsp. chopped fresh fennel leaves

Heat the oil in a deep sauté pan. Add the onions, shallots, fennel, and celery, and brown slightly on medium for a few minutes, turning so vegetable pieces are well coated in oil. Add the chicken stock, bring it to a boil, then reduce heat to low, and cover the pan. Let the ingredients simmer for 20 minutes. Remove the lid and taste the sauce. Season with sage and salt and pepper to taste. Add the walnuts, cover, and continue to cook the mixture, stirring every so often, for another 5 minutes. Add the mushrooms, cover, and stir the mixture every so often for another 10-12 minutes until mushrooms are done and walnuts have softened to your liking. Cut any vegetable pieces that seem too large. If there's extra liquid, remove cover and cook down to reduce liquid slightly (but leave some liquid for reheating). Add additional salt and pepper if needed. Keep covered on warm – or refrigerate and reheat the next day. Just before serving, sprinkle with chopped fresh parsley and fennel leaves. Makes seven 1/2-cup servings.

* Recipes reprinted from Healthier Holidays Going Against the Grain *E-book by Melissa Diane Smith.*

Chapter 13 – January:

Partying Gluten-Free Style

Feel like celebrating? Go ahead. There is a lot to celebrate these days! It's much more fun to socialize with others when you feel so much healthier without gluten in your diet. Plus, with the growing awareness in gluten-free eating and the wide variety of gluten-free foods now available, going to a party and eating gluten-free – or hosting a gluten-free party – is easier than ever.

Whether you're ringing in the New Year, attending a party, or throwing a football game bash, you can enjoy yourself without gluten – and few people will know or care about your special diet. Try these tips:

• **Make nibblies for people to nosh on.** Some examples: gluten-free meatballs in Italian pasta sauce, tail-on shrimp or steak tidbits sautéed in olive oil, gluten-free deli turkey slices, mini-chicken kabobs, garlic-sautéed mushrooms, assorted olives, nuts such as macadamia nuts or roasted almonds, Kaia Foods Kale Chips in several flavors, Blue Diamond Nut Thins with cheese slices or goat cheese, Mary's Gone Crackers rounds or Crunchmaster Original Multi-Seed Crackers with hummus, mini-fruit kabobs on party toothpicks, and vegetable crudités served with an Annie's gluten-free salad dressing. These are foods you can get together quickly and easily.

• **Transform a party into a fiesta with guacamole.**
Make a football gathering feel like a party by topping organic
burgers or turkey burgers (with or without cheese) with
avocado-based guacamole, which you can buy ready-to-eat or
easily make yourself. Serve the burgers on a small bed of lettuce
with sliced red onion and tomatoes, and have other items that
people can help themselves to: a bowl of roasted pistachios,
bowls of Lundberg Farms rice chips, Garden of Eatin' organic
non-GMO yellow corn or blue corn chips, lower-glycemic Bean
Brand Foods Beanitos bean chips, or Mexican-style flax
crackers with guacamole and salsa for dips, and sparkling
water, wine, or gluten-free beer, such as Anheuser-Busch
Redbridge or Bard's Tale Dragon's Gold.

• **Think ahead before going to a party.** To avoid taking
chances or accidentally eating something with gluten, it's best
to talk to the hostess several days before the party, tell her that
you are on a special diet, and politely ask what types of foods
will be served. If the hostess isn't knowledgeable or
accommodating, offer to bring a dish of your own – the main
way to be sure to avoid cross-contamination or inadvertent
mistakes with ingredients.

• **Bring an all-in-one dish.** When preparing a dish for
potlucks or parties, it's a good idea to make a dish that has meat
and vegetables together, with or without gluten-free grains.
Even if other foods aren't safe to eat, you can sustain yourself
with your dish that is a complete meal. Good all-in-one dishes

include: a big salad with broiled chicken strips, toasted pecans and pieces of apple; Spanish rice (with brown rice, meat, onions, tomato juice or tomato sauce, and cheese); Oriental chicken-vegetable stir-fries with gluten-free tamari sauce; and Shrimp-Spinach-Artichoke Salad (see recipe below).

• **Eat before the party.** If you didn't talk with the host ahead of time or bring your own dish, make sure to eat some protein, such as a baked chicken leg, turkey slices, or leftover pieces of pot roast, before you head to the party. It will give you staying power and keep you from getting so famished that you end up eating something you shouldn't. Then look for veggie sticks or fruit pieces to nibble on at the party. To enjoy yourself and feel well, it's always better to be safe than sorry.

Here's a colorful dish that is a real crowd pleaser at parties or potlucks. It's a ballpark recipe, meaning that you can add a bit more of this or that, depending on your preferences and tolerances, and it always comes out well.

Shrimp-Spinach-Artichoke Salad

1/3 cup organic extra virgin olive oil

1-lb. bag of jumbo, peeled shrimp with tail-on, thawed
6 to 10 thin asparagus spears, chopped into
   1-inch pieces
1-3 carrots, sliced
1/2 medium onion, chopped
1/4-1/2 red pepper, chopped (optional)
1 small shallot, chopped (optional)
1/2 cup chopped artichoke hearts or hearts of palm
3 to 6 garlic cloves, crushed and finely minced
4 to 6 cups fresh spinach leaves (stems removed,
   if desired)
2 to 3 Tbsp. chopped fresh parsley leaves (optional)
Oregano to taste (optional)
Ground coriander to taste (optional)
Unrefined sea salt and pepper to taste
Juice of 2 limes and 1 to 2 lemons

In a wok, add extra virgin olive oil and heat on medium. Sauté hard vegetables – such as carrot slices, chopped fresh asparagus, and chopped onion – for 4 to 6 minutes until they're almost done. (You can add chopped red pepper about halfway through, if you're using it). Add the shrimp and cook on one side until they turn pink, then turn each shrimp over and cook until pink on all sides. Then add the soft or quick-cooking vegetables: chopped shallot and garlic, artichoke hearts or sliced hearts of palm, and fresh spinach leaves. (The spinach shrinks when it cooks so add more than you think you need.) Add dried herbs and seasonings. Sauté until spinach is just barely cooked. Then take sautéed shrimp and veggies away from the burner and sprinkle with fresh parsley. You can serve this hot, but to make as a cold salad to take to parties, transfer to a room-temperature Pyrex (glass) container. Add fresh lemon juice and lime juice. Allow to cool. (At this stage, you can take tails off shrimp and cut the shrimp into pieces – or you can leave them whole. The shrimp with tails look elegant, but the shrimp pieces are easier to eat.) Once the mixture is room temperature, put lid on the glass container, and place in the refrigerator. The flavor is actually best half a day to a day-and-a-half later after marinating in the refrigerator. Taste before serving and add more lemon juice or herbs to taste if needed.

Variation with Kelp Noodles: Use 1/2 cup olive oil instead of 1/3 cup, follow above directions, then mix in 1/2 package Sea Tangle Kelp Noodles that have been cut into smaller pieces just before you put the lid on the container and place it in the refrigerator.

* *Recipe reprinted from Shrimp-Spinach-Artichoke Salad recipe in* Healthier Holidays Going Against the Grain *by Melissa Diane Smith.*

Chapter 14 – February:

Cold and Flu Protection and Relief

When it's cold and flu season, the last thing you want is to start to feel tired, achy, and chilled – or to develop a sore throat, cough, or the sniffles. No matter who you are, it is always difficult to take care of yourself but doubly challenging when you have gluten sensitivity. You have to find treatments that make you feel better, but also make sure every food and remedy that you take is free of gluten so you can boost your immunity, not hurt it, to fend off or overcome illness.

Be prepared. Stock up on essential gluten-free foods and remedies before you are sick so you can take them at the first sign of cold or flu symptoms. Try these tips:

• **Let garlic be your medicine.** Garlic has antiviral, antibacterial, and immune-boosting properties, and raw garlic is more therapeutic than cooked garlic. You can add a smashed and minced garlic clove into a vinegar- or lemon-juice-and olive oil salad dressing. Or mix minced garlic into a tablespoon of nut butter and eat it – a remedy I myself take when a sore throat is just starting to develop.

• **Make chicken soup**, a tried-and-true folk remedy. Sipping warm soup can make a sore throat feel better and the steam it provides can clear nasal passages, helping to relieve cold and flu symptoms. Additionally, sipping hot liquids can raise the temperature in the nose and throat above the threshold that cold and flu viruses can survive. Plus, chicken soup is simple to prepare, nutritious, and easily digested, making it a wonderful food for winter convalescents. To be on the safe side, always keep extra gluten-free chicken broth (i.e., Shelton's or Pacific Foods) stocked at your house. That way, if you can't make chicken soup from scratch, you can prepare a makeshift soup and receive some benefit quickly.

• **Drink other hot liquids** to warm up the body, help relieve nasal congestion, and soothe inflamed membranes that line your nose and throat. Green tea may be particularly effective at boosting immunity and preventing and reducing cold and flu symptoms. Need green tea without caffeine? Try Bigelow decaf green tea or Good Earth decaf green tea with lemongrass.

• **Try a gluten-free elderberry formulation**, such as Nature's Way Sambucus sugar-free black elderberry syrup. In folk medicine, flowers from the black elder bush were used to ease cold and flu symptoms and research with elderberry extract suggests it has antiviral and immune-boosting properties. One small study showed that 93 percent of flu patients given a standardized elderberry extract were completely symptom-free within two days, compared to those who took a placebo who recovered in about six days.

• **Consider protecting yourself with NAC,** especially if you are elderly or in a weakened condition and at high risk of developing the flu. N-acetyl cysteine (NAC) has antioxidant and immune-regulating properties and one study found that supplements of 600 mg NAC taken twice daily during flu season can dramatically reduce the frequency and severity of flu-like symptoms in elderly high-risk individuals. NAC supplements labeled gluten-free include those by Jarrow Formulas and Solgar.

• **Think zinc.** Several studies have found that zinc lozenges reduce the length and severity of cold symptoms. Gluten-free zinc lozenges include Cold-Eeze and Zand Herbal Formulas.

Feeling sick and rundown and don't feel like making Chicken Soup from scratch? Here's a shortcut to give you therapeutic Chicken Soup in a hurry. Based on how you feel, you can make it bland (by following the recipe) or add more flavor by making the variations.

Quick Chicken Soup

3 cups gluten-free chicken broth

1 large boneless chicken breast, cut
   into 1/2-inch pieces
1 large carrot, chopped
1 large celery stalk, chopped
1/4 to 1/2 small onion, chopped
2 to 3 garlic cloves, smashed and minced
2 Tbsp. fresh parsley leaves (optional)
Juice of 1/4 lemon per bowl (optional)

Heat the chicken broth in a pan on high until it starts to boil. Add the chicken breast pieces, carrot, celery and onion. When it starts to boil again, cover with lid, reduce heat to low, and simmer. After 7-8 minutes, add the garlic, simmer for a few more minutes, and add the parsley. Spoon into a bowl and eat as is or squeeze with lemon juice. Makes 4 bowls.

Variations:

- Add dried oregano leaves or rubbed sage and chopped shallot when you add the other ingredients, or add chopped fresh oregano or sage leaves when you add the garlic.

- To make Chicken-Rice or Chicken-Quinoa Soup, add cooked brown rice or cooked quinoa when you add the garlic.

- To make a Chicken-Noodle Soup, rinse, chop, and add Sea Tangle Kelp Noodles at the last minute.

- Add one-eighth of a jalapeno pepper and some diced tomatoes to simmer in the soup, then some fresh lime juice, sliced avocado, chopped fresh cilantro leaves, and crumbled, organic, non-GMO, white corn chips at the end to make a Quick Chicken Tortilla Soup.

* Recipe reprinted from Healthier Holidays Going Against the Grain E-book *by Melissa Diane Smith.*

Chapter 15 – March:

No Grains? No Problem!

Five years ago Vickie Laroue was diagnosed with celiac disease, autoimmune thyroid disease, and several heart-disease risk factors: high insulin levels, excess weight around the waistline, and high blood triglycerides. Going gluten free helped her digestive discomfort but it didn't solve the rest of her health problems. Over time, Vickie found that reducing her carb intake and avoiding all grains was a much more therapeutic diet prescription for her.

Grain-free eating is based mainly on meat and vegetables. Fortunately, newly available grain-free products, such as those that follow, can add much-needed convenience and variety to a diet that goes totally against the grain.

• **Kelp noodles.** A low-carb, low-calorie, pasta alternative is noodles made out of kelp by the Sea Tangle Noodle Company. Kelp is a sea vegetable that's rich in iodine and many other nutrients. Kelp noodles do not taste fishy but instead have a neutral taste that picks up the flavors of any food you combine with them. Try the noodles in salads or add them at the last minute to stir-fries or soups.

• **Raw food bars.** Quick-to-grab bars with the simplest of ingredients are date-based fruit and nut bars made by companies such as Larabar, Think Organic and Nature's Path

Organic. Made with uncooked ingredients, these bars are rich in fiber, nutrients and enzymes. However, they are not low carb – something low-carb dieters should beware of. The bars, which can make great, no-added-sugar "desserts," come in flavors as varied as Cherry Pie, Chocolate Coconut, and Chia Razz.

• **Flax-based crackers.** For a crunchy snack instead of rice-based crackers or corn-based chips, flax crackers by Foods Alive and Go Raw can fill the bill. Flax crackers are rich in fiber and also in omega-3 fatty acids, which are anti-inflammatory in nature and important in everything from heart health to reproductive health. These crackers come in plain varieties, and also savory varieties (such as Onion-Garlic), spicy varieties (such as Mexican and Italian Zest), and sweet varieties (such as Maple & Cinnamon and Banana "Bread").

• **Seed-based tortilla substitutes.** Raw Makery has developed a bendable, chewy and very tasty sprouted-flax-seed-based Rawtilla. To me, it tastes like a hearty bread. Just top this tortilla substitute with lettuce, meat and a condiment and fold it over to make a quick grain-free, nutrient-rich sandwich.

• **Nut flour.** Gluten-free baked goods made with rice flour and other gluten-free flours are high in carbohydrates and can lead to weight gain and worsened carbohydrate sensitivity. A solution is baked goods made with nut flours. They are lower in carbohydrates and are good sources of fiber and fat, so they stabilize blood sugar levels more than typical gluten-free flours. You can grind your own nut flour a quarter cup at a time in a blender using naturally low-carb nuts such as almonds, hazelnuts, pecans or walnuts. Or you can buy ready-to-use almond meal, a heavier flour, by NOW Foods or Trader Joe's, or blanched almond flour, a lighter flour, by companies such as Dowd & Rogers and Bob's Red Mill. Nut flours add texture, richness and flavor to baked goods and are good sources of vitamin E, magnesium, fiber, and heart-healthy monounsaturated fats. Another benefit: Studies show that eating nuts regularly reduces the risk of heart disease, diabetes and macular degeneration.

• **Coconut flour.** Another grain-free, low-carb flour alternative is coconut flour, made by various companies including Bob's Red Mill. Coconut flour has a unique nutritional benefit: It has far more blood-sugar-balancing and help-you-feel-full fiber than any other flour. When used by itself, coconut flour produces baked goods that are light, fluffy and moist. But because of its sky-high fiber content, it performs differently than all other flours, so it's best to follow recipes designed specifically for coconut flour until you become accustomed to working with it. Try recipes in *Cooking with Coconut Flour* by Bruce Fife, ND, but adapt them to eliminate the sugar.

Many people who avoid grains avoid sugar, too. Here's an easy-to-make, grain-free muffin recipe that is sweetened with just fruit for people on low-carb or no-added-sugar diets. These muffins don't taste very sweet right out of the oven but the flavor improves and becomes sweeter when the muffins are refrigerated. When using liquefied coconut oil in baking, always make sure that all other ingredients that you use, including the eggs, are room temperature.

Banana-Coconut Muffins

3 eggs

2 Tbsp. coconut oil

1/3 cup mashed banana (about 1 small ripe banana)

1 tsp. Frontier Herbs alcohol-free vanilla flavor or
   vanilla extract

1/4 tsp. unrefined sea salt

1/4 cup coconut flour

1 Tbsp. almond meal or hazelnut flour

1/4 tsp. Featherweight baking powder

1/2 tsp. ground cinnamon

1 Tbsp. shredded coconut

2 Tbsp. raisins (optional)

Preheat oven to 400 degrees. Melt coconut oil if it is not liquefied. Make sure the other ingredients are at room temperature. Mix together the first five ingredients. Add the coconut flour, almond or hazelnut flour, baking powder, cinnamon, and shredded coconut, and whisk together until smooth. Fold in raisins if using. Pour into muffin cups that have been greased with coconut oil. Bake at 400 degrees for 15 minutes or until a toothpick inserted in a muffin comes out clean. Pop muffins onto a wire rack to cool, then store in a container and refrigerate. Flavor is best one or two days after baking. Makes 6 muffins.

Chapter 16 – April:

Gluten Free and Eco-Friendly

When Suzy Schuster began eating gluten free eight years ago, all she cared about was making sure the foods she ate had no gluten. That seemed like a tall task at first, but over time it became easier and easier. Today it is second nature.

As Suzy became increasingly comfortable with gluten-free eating, she gradually became more informed about the food she ate and started to realize there was another food issue that was important to her: choosing foods that were better for the environment. Difficult as it might have seemed before she began changing her diet so dramatically, she found there were easy ways to select gluten-free foods that were good for her health and good for the planet.

In celebration of Earth Day, try these tips to choose eco-friendly foods that have a low impact on the environment:

• **Buy organic.** Although it seems counterintuitive, conventional farming today uses petrochemical pesticides and fertilizers in the growing of crops. The pesticides harm numerous species of beneficial insects, butterflies, and birds. Excessive use of chemical fertilizers contaminates our water. And the production, transportation and application of synthetic pesticides and fertilizers are energy-intensive and use a lot of fossil fuel. When you buy fruits, vegetables, gluten-free grains, and other foods with "Certified Organic" seals on them, it means they were grown without using most conventional pesticides or synthetic fertilizers. That in turn means less energy or fossil fuel is used in producing them.

- **Go for no GMOs.** The five major genetically modified organism (GMO) foods – corn, soy, cottonseed, canola and sugar beets – are gene-spliced to either tolerate chemical herbicides, or produce chemical insectides. To do your part for better planet health, steer clear of foods made with these five ingredients unless they are labeled certified organic or non-GMO. To learn more, visit the non-GMO website, NonGMOShoppingGuide.com.

- **Seek out locally grown foods.** The average fresh food product on our dinner table travels 1,500 miles to get there. Buying locally produced food (or growing some vegetables on your own) eliminates fuel-guzzling transportation costs and helps conserve our limited fuel resources.

- **Choose more grass-fed meats.** Commercial meat production involves fattening cattle on commercially grown corn, and the production of large amounts of corn feed uses high amounts of chemical pesticides and fertilizers and therefore more oil and natural gas. Raising grass-fed cattle eliminates those chemicals and costs, helping save our oil and gas for better uses.

• **Try a more eco-friendly rice.** There has been a breakthrough in producing rice – the System of Rice Intensification (SRI), a set of ecologically sound concepts and practices that change the way rice is typically grown. SRI methods were developed in Madagascar in the early 1980s and have spread to over 35 countries with the help of many organizations, including Cornell University. The innovative methods enable farmers with limited resources to increase their rice yields using 80 to 90 percent less seed, 25 to 50 percent less water, and few or no chemical fertilizers and pesticides. And the farmers are able to use seeds of the traditional varieties of rice they have historically grown. To help support this cause, try the three types of SRI-grown rice available from Lotus Foods: Cambodian Flower Rice, Madagascar Pink Rice, and Indonesian Volcano Rice. By following one or more of these tips, we all can play a part in producing a healthier food system and a healthier planet.

This rice pilaf is made with SRI-grown Madagascar Pink Rice and organic and locally grown ingredients. It takes only 25 minutes to make, is a nice addition to an Easter meal, and goes well with most meat, poultry, fish, and vegetarian entrees. If you're carbohydrate sensitive or grain sensitive, forgo the rice and serve Roasted Asparagus and Mushrooms. They're delicious all on their own.

Pink Rice Pilaf with Roasted Asparagus and Mushrooms

1 cup Lotus Foods Madagascar Pink Rice
1-1/2 cups gluten-free organic or homemade
  chicken broth
1-1/2 cups locally grown thin asparagus cut into
   1- to 1-1/2-inch pieces (woody ends removed)
8 oz. organic sliced mushrooms
1 small organic garlic clove, crushed and minced
3 Tbsp. organic extra virgin olive oil
1 Tbsp. organic butter (or organic extra virgin
  olive oil as a dairy-free alternative)
Unrefined sea salt to taste
Juice of 1/4 lemon (optional)
1 Tbsp. chopped locally grown organic parsley

Bring broth and rice to a boil in a pan. Cover, reduce heat, and simmer 20 minutes. Preheat oven to 400 degrees. Once the rice starts simmering, put asparagus pieces, mushroom slices, and minced garlic in a bowl. Add oil and mix well to evenly coat. Spread asparagus mixture in a single layer on a cookie sheet lightly oiled with olive oil, pouring any remaining oil and garlic over all. Roast 15-18 minutes, until tender. Add the roasted vegetables into the rice, and mix in butter, optional lemon juice, and sea salt to taste. Sprinkle with chopped fresh parsley, and serve. Makes six 1/2-cup servings.

Chapter 17 – May:

Getting Enough Fiber
on a Gluten-Free Diet

We've been repeatedly told that whole grains are good sources of fiber and that fiber has many health benefits: It keeps our bowels working regularly, prevents constipation, helps us feel full, reduces cholesterol levels and helps control blood sugar levels.

But if you follow a gluten-free diet and cut wheat, rye, barley and even oats out of your diet, can you get enough of the fiber you need to keep yourself healthy? The answer is unequivocally yes – and you can do so in lots of tasty ways. Try these tips:

• **Eat like a caveman.** It may seem hard to believe but you can get more than enough fiber eating vegetables, fruits, nuts and seeds. The problem is most Americans are not in the habit of eating many fruits and vegetables so they don't get enough when they switch to a gluten-free diet. If you do a gluten-free or grain-free diet the right way – by replacing grain products with plenty of fresh fruits and vegetables – it's easy to get sufficient fiber. A 2002 analysis found that a grain-free, meat-containing Stone Age or Paleolithic sample diet can provide 42.5 grams of dietary fiber per day, considerably higher than the 15 grams found in the standard U.S. diet and the recommended daily fiber amount of 25-30 grams. So, load up on salads, raw vegetable sticks and steamed or cooked vegetables – and eat fresh fruit instead of drinking fruit juice. Strive for a total of five to nine servings of vegetables and fruits each day. Especially good vegetable and fruit fiber sources are artichokes and artichoke hearts, broccoli, carrots, raspberries, blackberries, and pears and apples with their skins on.

• **Go a bit nutty.** Nuts are rich in both fiber and flavor, so use them in lots of different ways. Snack on various kinds, use them in baking, and add them to salads and cooked vegetables. Also try coconut, another high-fiber source: Sprinkle dried shredded coconut on fresh fruit or gluten-free cereal, and use coconut flour to make muffins and quick breads.

• **Try dried fruit.** If you have a tendency toward constipation, include more dried fruit in your diet. Dried figs, dried plums (prunes), dates and date-based fruit bars such as Larabar are all good choices, supplying 3 to 5 grams of fiber per serving.

• **Slowly add other high-fiber foods.** Experiment with legumes (i.e., split peas, chickpeas, lentils, pinto beans, black beans, and red kidney beans) and gluten-free whole grains (i.e., brown rice, wild rice, quinoa, buckwheat groats, amaranth and teff). Other fiber-rich foods include butternut or acorn squash, sweet potatoes and yams, flaxseed and flaxseed crackers, and easy-to-fix Perky's Nutty Flax or Ruth's Chia Goodness cereal. As health enhancing as fiber is, it's important to *gradually* add fiber to your diet and to drink a lot of water. A rapid increase in fiber can cause stomach and intestinal distress, including gas, bloating and diarrhea – conditions that mimic common reactions to gluten.

• **Dig into avocado.** An easy, fun way to get extra fiber is to add sliced avocado or a scoop of avocado-based guacamole to a salad or entrée. It may surprise you, but avocados have the highest fiber content of any fruit.

This recipe is versatile, easy to make, and chock-full of fiber from many different sources. Plus, you can make it in lots of different ways based on what ingredients you have on hand.

Melissa's Quick High-Fiber Muesli

1/2 medium organic apple with the skin on, chopped
2 Tbsp. chopped pecans or walnuts
1 Tbsp. raisins
1/2 tsp. ground cinnamon
3 Tbsp. Perky's Nutty Flax Cereal or 3 Tbsp. cooked
    red quinoa or 1 Tbsp. almond flour (optional)
1/4 cup coconut milk

1 Tbsp. dried shredded coconut

1-1/2 tsp. ground flaxseed (optional)

In a bowl, mix together the chopped apple, nuts, raisins, cinnamon and optional cereal, quinoa or almond flour if using. Pour coconut milk over the mixture, stir to distribute the coconut milk, and let it sit for 5 minutes. Add a teaspoon or two of water if you prefer a wetter consistency. Sprinkle shredded coconut and optional ground flaxseed on top. Serves 1. Recipe can be doubled, tripled or quadrupled as needed.

Variations:

- Add 1/2 medium chopped pear, 1 chopped nectarine or 3/4 cup blueberries, blackberries, raspberries or strawberries in place of the apple.

- Add slivered almonds or hazelnut pieces in place of the walnuts or pecans.

Chapter 18 – June:

Making Your Summer a Picnic

One of the special joys of warm weather is eating outdoors. Whether you grab a brown-bag lunch by yourself, have a family gathering at a picnic table, or enjoy a spread of elegant food for two on a blanket, make this time of year a gluten-free picnic. Try these tips:

• **Prepare sandwiches or wraps for impromptu picnics.** If you don't have much time, use gluten-free bread (i.e., Food for Life Bhutanese Red Rice Bread), organic corn tortillas, or Raw Makery Rawtillas with gluten-free fillings (nut butter or Applegate Farms lunch meats) to make nut butter, turkey, roast beef, or ham and cheese sandwiches in a jiffy. Throw in a pack of celery or carrot sticks, an apple, and a gluten-free, date-based fruit-and-nut bar (such as a Larabar or a Think Organic! bar) for a brown bag full of satisfying food that you can put together in ten minutes or less.

• **Use salads as main dishes, side dishes or desserts.** When you have more time to plan foods to carry in a cooler, put on your thinking cap and get creative with salads. For side salads, try potato salad, quinoa-based tabouli, or assorted veggies marinated in gluten-free vinaigrette dressing. For main dish salads, make green salads with lettuce, assorted vegetables, and chilled cooked steak, chicken or fish. Bring a gluten-free salad dressing in a container to pour on at the last minute. Or create main-dish pasta salads with meat or shrimp, ingredients such as chopped olives, hearts of palm, or artichoke hearts, and gluten-free rice pasta or Sea Tangle Kelp Noodles. For dessert, make colorful, assorted fruit salads, such as blueberries, raspberries and sliced strawberries; sliced nectarines and pitted, halved Bing cherries; or fresh pineapple cubes topped with shredded coconut.

• **Put together a spread of finger food.** Picnics don't have to be elaborate. Sometimes the most fun of all is nibbling on assorted finger food in between good conversation or breaks for throwing a Frisbee or football back and forth. Bring guacamole, salsa or hummus with organic blue corn chips, Mexican- or Italian-style flax crackers, assorted raw veggie sticks, and chilled cooked tail-on shrimp. Other foods to nosh on: Gluten-free cold cuts or slices of cheese. Garlic-stuffed olives. Bags of almonds or Macadamia nuts. Kaia Foods Sea Salt & Vinegar Kale Chips. Red or green grapes. Savory sprouted sunflower seeds, or trail mixes, such as Enjoy Life Foods Beach Bash, a collection of seeds and sulfite-free dried fruits.

• **Re-use your meat leftovers.** Slices of cold pot roast meat, roast chicken, or roast turkey breast meat all work nicely at picnics. So do cold cooked meat kabob cubes or fajita meat strips. You can also combine leftover cooked chicken, turkey or fish with chopped celery, onion and gluten-free mayonnaise (i.e., Spectrum Naturals Organic Olive Oil Mayonnaise) to make chicken, turkey or fish salad. Then use that salad as a filling inside sandwiches or on top of lettuce greens.

A refreshing, healthier, lighter alternative to traditional mayonnaise-based potato salad, this is a great side dish to take to a picnic.

Greek Potato Salad

2 lbs. medium-sized red potatoes
6 Tbsp. organic extra virgin olive oil
4 Tbsp. fresh lemon juice
3/4 cup chopped white or yellow onion
1/2 cup chopped fresh parsley
Unrefined sea salt and pepper to taste
Additional fresh lemon juice to taste (optional)

Scrub potatoes and quarter them. Put the potatoes in a large saucepan, add water to cover potatoes by at least 1 inch of water, and add a pinch of salt. Cover and bring to a boil. Simmer over medium-low heat until a fork can pierce the center of the largest potato easily, about 15 to 20 minutes. While the potatoes cook, chop the onion and the parsley and make the dressing by mixing the olive oil, lemon juice and salt and pepper to taste. When the potatoes are done, drain them, and use a fork or knife to peel off the skins. Place them in a non-metallic serving bowl or dish, and cut large potato pieces in half. Add onions and parsley and pour on the dressing. Using a large fork and spoon, toss the salad and keep mixing until all the dressing is well distributed and absorbed into the potato salad. Cover and refrigerate for at least a few hours or preferably overnight for the flavors to meld. Before heading to your picnic, mix well, taste, and add more salt or lemon juice if needed. Makes seven 1/2-cup servings.

Chapter 19 – July:

Enjoying the Juicy Fruits of Summer

During uncomfortably hot summer days, there is nothing quite as refreshing as naturally sweet, moisture-rich fruit. Packed with nutrients, fiber and water, fruit is nature's antidote to rising outdoor temperatures. It also is a special bonus of summer: There are more types of fresh fruit in season, which means more luscious flavors and vibrant colors to play with when making meals, snacks, and desserts. Use the bounty of fresh fruit to its fullest to add new life to regular gluten-free fare. Try these tips to enjoy fruit in many tasty ways:

• **Eat whole or sliced fruit as is.** The simplest way to eat fruit is to grab it and eat it, or pack it and eat it later. In-season fruits that work especially well as grab-and-go snacks are plums and nectarines. Fruits that make festive additions to a 4th of July get-together are fresh raspberries, cherries, or sliced watermelon.

• **Create fruit salads.** Summer fruits taste delicious on their own, but you can make them even more special by mixing them in different combinations to make a wide variety of fruit salads. Get a variety of your favorite fruits, chop them and combine together. It's a simple formula that yields wonderful results for your labor. Combinations to try include: assorted melons, berries and grapes; or peaches, apples, pineapple, banana and coconut; or nectarines, plums, blueberries and pitted, halved cherries. Serve in a colorful or clear glass bowl, or for a special party presentation, spoon freshly made fruit salad into a scooped-out watermelon, melon, or pineapple boat.

- **Fix fruit with "cream".** For an easy sugar-free treat, pour organic whipping cream or half and half over fresh strawberries or sliced peaches. If you avoid dairy, use an alternative to milk, such as Blue Diamond Unsweetened Vanilla Almond Breeze. Or make your own substitute cream with organic coconut milk mixed to taste with several drops of Frontier Herbs' alcohol-free vanilla flavor.

- **Serve pancakes topped with fruit.** For a special addition to breakfast or brunch, make pancakes out of the gluten-free flour of your choice (i.e., brown rice flour, sorghum flour, millet flour, quinoa flour, amaranth flour, chestnut flour, coconut flour, or almond meal or flour) and top them with fresh berries or sliced nectarines.

- **Add fruit to green salads.** Fruit brings a bright flavor surprise to side salads or main-dish salads. In romaine, green leaf, mixed baby green, or spinach salads, try tossing in raspberries, sliced strawberries, chopped peaches, pears, apples, grapes, or pitted, halved cherries, with other ingredients such as shredded carrot, jicama sticks, toasted nuts, chopped avocado, chopped hard-boiled egg, or crumbled goat cheese.

- **Try fruit salsa on entrees.** To add a refreshing, almost party-like feel to cooked fish, poultry or pork, make fruit salsa by combining chopped fruit with onion, chives, green onions or shallots, different types of peppers, tomato and lime juice if desired, and fresh cilantro. Tropical fruits, such as pineapple, papaya or mango, are the most common fruits used in fruit salsa, but fresh peaches, strawberries, or cherries also can be used.

Adding fresh fruit to a main-dish salad is refreshing for lunch or dinner on a hot summer day. This salad is easy enough to make that it can be regular fare during the summer but it's tasty enough to serve guests. You can also eliminate the chicken or turkey and serve it as a side salad for four people.

Chicken and Strawberry Salad with Cilantro-Lime Dressing

1/4 cup chopped pecans
3 to 3-1/2 cups organic romaine lettuce or mixed
    baby greens
1/4 cup shredded carrot
1/2 cup sliced hulled fresh organic strawberries

5 cooked chicken strips or 2/3 cup cubed or
chopped turkey breast
4 jicama sticks or 4 hearts of palm, chopped
(optional)

1/2 cup packed fresh cilantro leaves
1/4 cup organic extra virgin olive oil
1-1/2 Tbsp. fresh lime juice
1-1/2 Tbsp. fresh orange juice
1/4 tsp. unrefined sea salt
Black pepper to taste (optional)

Toast nuts in a 325-degree oven for 5 to 7 minutes until fragrant. Puree the ingredients for the dressing in a blender. Put the lettuce on two plates, add the additional toppings on top of the greens, and drizzle the dressing on top of each salad. Serves 2.

Chapter 20 – August:

Making You Own Fast Food

Busy and short on time? That happens to all of us and, when it does, it's natural to want to cut corners and grab fast food. Unfortunately, eating most commercial fast food is a quick way to become ill, whether from the hidden gluten or from the excessive amounts of salt, sugar and unhealthy fats and meats. Some people who are in a hurry heat up gluten-free frozen meals, but most frozen meals aren't very tasty, and they are expensive and too high in salt and carbohydrates for good health for most people.

To successfully maneuver through the busiest times in our lives, it's important to provide well-balanced nutrition in the simplest possible ways to keep us going strong. Try these tips for making quick and healthy meals:

• **Prepare tasty pieces of meat.** Take less than thirty minutes to fix batches of protein that you can use to create future meals. You can broil up chicken strips (see recipe at the end of this chapter); chicken, lamb, pork, beef or shrimp kabobs; turkey burgers, lamb burgers or grass-fed hamburgers; or lamb chops or steaks. Eat some of the meat with vegetables for a meal at the time you cook it, then chop up the leftover meat and refrigerate it to use as a base ingredient when making future meals.

- **Combine the meat with vegetables for fast food.** Add the meat, either cold or reheated, to salads with assorted vegetables, or reheat the meat at the same time you cook some vegetables, such as green beans, broccoli, or asparagus and mushrooms. Both types of meals take less than ten minutes to make.

- **Make meat and vegetable combinations.** If you have time off on the weekend, make a hearty meal such as a pot roast with carrots, onions, green beans and a potato or two, or use a Crock-Pot to make the meal while you're away during the day. Save the leftovers in the fridge and reheat them for a balanced fast meal in a day or so – or freeze them and have them a week later. Another easy meat-and-vegetable combination dish to make is a stir-fry. Just heat macadamia nut oil or coconut oil in a wok, add shrimp or chicken or pork stir-fry strips, and toss in a bunch of vegetables, such as the pack of fresh Chinese stir-fry vegetables sold at Trader Joe's, with garlic and/or ginger, and sea salt or Bragg's Liquid Amino Acids. This is another dish that takes less than ten minutes to make and is quick and easy to reheat.

- **Add a little grain if needed.** It's certainly not necessary, but you can add gluten-free grains to the basic meat-and-vegetable combinations above if you desire. Some of the quickest and most nutritious grains to fix are Organic Sunshine Burgers, including its Garden Herb and new Falafel variety, which take a little more than ten minutes to make; Ancient

Harvest Original or Inca Red Quinoa, which cooks in 15 minutes; and Lotus Foods Bhutanese Red Rice or Madagascar Pink Rice, which cooks in 20 minutes. Once you cook up grains, you can have them in the fridge to use with meat and vegetables to make quick meals, such as Savory Quinoa Hash (see recipe in Chapter 1), a day or two later.

• **Better yet, add more vegetables or some fruit or nuts.** As mentioned throughout this book, all of us should be eating more vegetables for better health. So, when you're reheating meat and cooking up one type of vegetable, try cooking up another type, or making a salad, or chopping some vegetables into vegetable sticks, so that you have double or triple the amount of vegetables to meat. This is quicker than making grain side dishes and better for your waistline. You can also finish your meal with some fruit, such as an apple or a bowl of berries. Or for additional concentrated calories, top your salad or vegetables with nuts. We tend to forget it, but vegetables, fruit and nuts are all healthy fast food.

Get in the habit of simply preparing tasty pieces of meat that you can use in handy ways in future meals and snacks. I often make these chicken strips as a staple fast food. I use them in salads, reheat them and eat them with cooked vegetables or brown or wild rice, and add them to soups.

Herbes de Provence Chicken Strips

1/4 cup Whole Foods Herbes de Provence Vinaigrette
2 Tbsp. organic extra virgin olive oil
Juice of half a lemon
1 lb. boneless chicken breast stir-fry strips

Mix the marinade ingredients together in a medium non-metallic bowl. Mix in the chicken strips and allow them to sit in the marinade for five minutes. Preheat your oven broiler to 450 degrees. Cover the bottom part of a small broiling pan with aluminum foil (for easy cleanup later), then put the rack of the broiling pan on top. Arrange the chicken strips on the broiling pan rack. Broil on the second-to-the-lowest rack in the oven for 8 to 10 minutes (depending on the size of the chicken strips), flip each piece over, and broil the other side. Serves 4.

Chapter 21 – September:

Going Nuts with Your Diet

Looking for a way to make your diet richer in nutrients and flavor? Try using more of nature's nutritional powerhouses, nuts and seeds. They carry all the ingredients necessary to nourish and sustain new plants, which makes them tiny morsels that pack amazingly big nutritional punches. This chapter gives a rundown on nuts. The next chapter covers seeds.

Research shows that eating nuts regularly in the diet confers many health benefits, including reducing the risk of type 2 diabetes, cardiovascular disease, sudden cardiac death, and macular degeneration. They're also rich in fiber, vitamin E and various minerals, such as heart-healthy potassium and magnesium. Yet people often avoid nuts because they think they're fattening. Studies suggest otherwise: People actually lose weight better on nut-rich diets, and those who eat nuts are leaner than those who don't.

If you find yourself bingeing on nuts, consider the possibility that you may have an allergy-addiction to a certain type of nut. Nuts are a common food allergen, so be sure to avoid any you are sensitive to. If you're allergic to one type, try others. There are many different food families of nuts.

Try these ways to incorporate more nuts into your diet:

- **Eat nuts as snacks.** A source of fat, protein, carbs and fiber, nuts make good mini-meals that help satisfy the appetite and stabilize lagging blood sugar levels in between meals. Carry almonds or Brazil nuts in your coat pocket, purse or briefcase to nosh on when you need them. Or serve macadamia nuts, peanuts (which are technically not nuts, but legumes), or pistachios at parties. Choose either raw or dry roasted without any other ingredients, or for a special treat, try Living Intentions gourmet- seasoned Gone Nuts! nut blends. You also can make your own home-toasted nuts by toasting raw nuts in your oven at home. If you're carbohydrate-sensitive, beware of cashews: they're the highest-carb nut next to chestnuts.

- **Use nuts as toppers or key ingredients.** Small amounts of nuts on top of or mixed into vegetable dishes, salads, or stir-fries can give regular fare gourmet flavor. Think green beans almondine, Waldorf salad (with walnuts, apples and celery), stuffing with pecans or walnuts, Chinese stir-fries with cashews, or Mediterranean vegetable sautés with pine nuts.

- **Spread nut butter around.** Almond butter and peanut butter are the two most common types, but cashew butter and cashew-macadamia butter are available, too. Some companies, such as Artisana and Futters Nut Butters, make pecan butter and walnut butter, too. You can try different types of nut butter for variety in your diet and spread them on gluten-free bread or crackers, apple slices, or celery sticks as snacks or a quick breakfast.

• **Bake with nut flour.** If you are sensitive to grains or simply want a substitute for rice flour from time to time, almond flour (available from many companies) and hazelnut flour (available from Bob's Red Mill) are two alternatives. You also can make your own flour with other nuts, such as pecans or walnuts, by grinding 1/4 cup of raw nuts at a time in a blender. For people who have diverticulitis – an intestinal condition characterized by inflamed pouches in the intestinal wall that can get aggravated by pieces of nuts – ground nuts can be a good alternative. Try sprinkling ground nuts on gluten-free cereals or salads.

Here is a nut-based baked good that serves nicely as a snack, an hors d'oeuvre topped with olive tapenade, or an accompaniment to soup or salad.

Savory Pecan Flatbread Rounds

1-1/2 cups blanched almond flour
3/4 tsp. Herbamare herb seasoning salt

1/2 tsp. gluten-free onion powder
1/4 tsp. ground thyme
1/2 cup very finely chopped pecans
1 large egg
1 Tbsp. organic extra virgin olive oil or
macadamia nut oil

In a large mixing bowl, stir together the almond flour, salt, onion powder, thyme and pecans. In a smaller bowl, whisk the egg a few minutes until frothy. Add in the oil and whisk again. Pour the liquid mixture into the dry ingredients and stir until the dough is well blended. Line a 10" x 14" stainless steel baking sheet with parchment paper. Drop dough by heaping tablespoon on the parchment paper allowing at least 1-1/2 inches between each mound. Cut another piece of parchment paper and place it over the mounds of dough. With a rolling pin or other cylindrical object, roll the mounds of dough out between the two pieces of parchment paper so that each one is roughly 1/8-inch thick. Remove the top piece of parchment paper. Round out edges of each round with your hands. Bake at 350 degrees for 10 minutes. Use a spatula to flip each cracker over, allow to cool, and serve or store. Makes 15 flatbread rounds. Recipe can be doubled for a larger batch.

If you don't tolerate eggs without adverse symptoms, you're not alone. Intolerance to eggs is quite common among people who are gluten sensitive.

While it is harder to bake without eggs, it is not impossible. As an alternative to the previous nut-flour-based flatbread recipe, here is a nut-flour-based cracker recipe without eggs. The two recipes are similar, except I used oil and water in place of the egg, which makes more of a cracker-like consistency instead of a flatbread consistency. It's still very good. You can create different versions by removing the caraway seeds and using other herbs.

Egg-Free Caraway Nut Crackers

1 cup blanched almond flour
1/2 cup hazelnut flour
1/2 tsp. Real Salt or Celtic salt
1/4 cup very finely chopped pecans
1/4 cup organic extra virgin olive oil or macadamia
   nut oil
1/4 cup water
1-1/2 tsp. caraway seeds (optional - for a "rye"-like
   flavor)

In a large mixing bowl, stir together the almond flour, hazelnut flour, salt, pecans, and caraway seeds. In a smaller bowl, mix the oil and water. Pour the liquid mixture into the dry ingredients and stir until the dough is well blended. Line a stainless steel baking sheet with parchment paper. Drop dough by heaping tablespoon on the parchment paper allowing at least 1-1/2 inches between each mound. Cut another piece of parchment paper and place it over the mounds of dough. With a rolling pin or other cylindrical object, roll the mounds of dough out between the two pieces of parchment paper so that each one is roughly 1/8-inch thick. Remove the top piece of parchment paper. Round out edges of each round with your hands. Bake at 350 degrees for 15 minutes or until cooked to desired crispness. Use a spatula to flip each cracker over, allow to cool, and serve or store. Makes 15 flatbread rounds. Recipe can be doubled for a larger batch.

Chapter 22 – October:

Planting New Seeds in Your Diet

If you're looking for an alternative to nuts or a simple way to get more nutrients in your gluten-free diet, look no further than seeds. Unlike nuts, seeds aren't common allergens, so they are better tolerated by people with food sensitivities. Plus, several seeds are rich in hard-to-get nutrients, such as omega-3 essential fatty acids, making them desirable even for people who don't have allergies.

The seeds people are most familiar with are sunflower seeds and pumpkin seeds, good seeds to snack on, and sesame seeds, which make nice additions to stir-fries and breadings. Flax seeds are well-known sources of omega-3s, which have anti-inflammatory properties but are notoriously low in the American diet. However, whole flax seeds tend to pass through the system undigested, so to get the most out of flaxseed without digestive distress, it's best to grind whole flax seeds before sprinkling on food.

Newer seeds on the market are hemp seeds and chia seeds, including Salba, a trademarked version of chia seed. Hulled or shelled hemp seeds, available from Bob's Red Mill, Manitoba Harvest, Nutiva, and Ruth's, are soft and easier to digest for people with digestive problems. They have a good balance of omega-6 to omega-3 fatty acids and are one of the few food sources of gamma-linolenic acid (GLA), another anti-inflammatory fat that many people take in supplement form.

Hemp seeds also are rich in fiber and have complete protein with all the essential amino acids.

Chia seeds are a member of the mint family and were used as a highly valued food in the Aztec diet. They are easily digestible but have such high fiber levels and can absorb so much water that they help release carbohydrates slowly into the bloodstream and may help to reduce cravings. They're also packed with nutrients. Two tablespoons of Salba, for example, provide 8 grams of fiber, 5 grams of protein, 184 mg of calcium and a whopping 5 grams of omega-3 fatty acids.

Try these ways to include more nutrient-rich seeds in your diet:

• **Sprinkle seeds on salads, fruit or yogurt.** Try hemp seeds in quinoa tabouli, sunflower seeds on salads, or black chia seeds, such as Ruth's Raw Goodness, mixed into yogurt or coconut milk with fruit.

• **Eat some seedy cereal.** Top your favorite gluten-free hot or cold cereal with a tablespoon of one type or a combination of seeds. Or try a seed-based cereal, such as Perky's Crunchy Flax, Ruth's Chia Goodness, Kaia Foods Buckwheat Granola, or Lydia's Organics Berry Good Cereal (made with sprouted sunflower seeds and sprouted flax). For lunch or dinner, try Hodgson Mill brown rice pasta with golden milled flax seed.

- **Snack on seeds.** Eat one type alone or make your own seed trail mixes. For a treat, splurge on Enjoy Life Foods Beach Bash or Mountain Mambo seed-and-dried-fruit trail mix.

- **Try sprouted seed products,** which are easier to digest for many people. Sprouted flaxseed crackers in a variety of flavors are available from Foods Alive and Go Raw, and Kaia Foods makes several tasty varieties of sprouted sunflower seeds, such as Garlic & Sea Salt and Sweet Curry. If you like to make food yourself, buy a dehydrator and make your own sprouted seed crackers.

- **Use seed butter as a spread.** If you are allergic to peanut butter or other nut butters, roasted organic SunButter sunflower butter, which is made in a nut-free facility, is a good substitute. Try it spread on gluten-free bread, crackers or celery sticks. Sesame tahini works well when making hummus or sauces, and a nutritious new seed butter to try is hemp seed butter, which has a light, nutty taste.

Having trouble trying to work more vegetables into your diet? Try this quick and tasty way to fix cauliflower with a seed-based sauce. The sauce tastes good on fish, too.

Cauliflower with Lemon-Tahini Sauce

1 small head cauliflower cut into florets
1/4 cup sesame tahini
1/2 tsp. organic gluten-free garlic powder
1/4 tsp. unrefined sea salt
1 Tbsp. organic extra virgin olive oil
1 Tbsp. lemon juice
1 Tbsp. water
2-3 tsp. chopped fresh organic parsley (optional)

Steam cauliflower 9 to 10 minutes until tender to your liking. While the cauliflower is cooking, mix the tahini, garlic powder and salt together in a coffee cup with a spoon until there are no lumps. Mix in the olive oil, then the lemon juice, then the water. Allow the sauce to sit for a few minutes, mix it again and check it, and add a tablespoon more water if you desire a thinner sauce. Spoon the cauliflower onto serving plates and spoon the sauce over the cauliflower. Top with chopped parsley. Serves 4.

Variation: For a more exotic taste, sprinkle with a shake or two of ground sumac, a Middle Eastern spice.

Chapter 23 – November:

Further Against the Grain: Going Paleo

Two years ago Cindy Armstrong went through the difficult process of learning to eat gluten free. Changing her diet lessened her digestive bloating but didn't reduce her heavy waistline or prediabetic blood sugar levels. Over time she also realized that other foods, such as soy, dairy products and non-gluten grains, caused digestive upset, and that eating sugar or other types of sweeteners triggered insatiable cravings and binge-eating.

"I wasn't feeling well and wasn't in control of my eating habits. I finally got to the point where I wanted to do something more drastic to help myself," Cindy remembers. "My nutritionist told me about the Paleolithic or hunter-gatherer diet – just going back to eating the types of foods our earliest ancestors evolved on and thrived on. It made sense, so I tried it. It turned out to be the answer I was looking for to stop my food cravings, clear up my digestive problems, and get my weight and blood sugar levels under control."

Also known as the Stone Age Diet, the Paleolithic diet is effective at reducing waist sizes and lowering blood sugar levels in people with heart disease and type 2 diabetes or other blood sugar problems, and it improves a wide range of cardiovascular risk factors in healthy, sedentary people in as little as ten days, according to recent research.

By taking gluten out of your diet, you already have taken an important step to eating Paleo. Here are more tips to help convert your diet:

- **Beef up on animal protein and veggies.** A central feature of a hunter-gatherer-type diet is high-quality, unprocessed animal protein – such as lean, organic, or grass-fed meats, wild-caught fish, and omega-3-enriched eggs – at every meal, surrounded by plentiful non-starchy vegetables, such as salad greens, artichoke, asparagus, broccoli, and zucchini. Starchy vegetables, such as yams, winter squash and sweet potatoes, should be avoided, but carrots are allowed and, in one study, limited quantities of potatoes were allowed without detriment.

- **Go *completely* against the grain.** Instead of just staying away from gluten, steer clear of all grains and grain-like foods – including oats, corn, millet, rice, sorghum, wild rice, amaranth, buckwheat, and quinoa. Also eliminate legumes (beans and peas). To do this, replace the gluten-free grains and beans you were eating in your diet with more servings of non-starchy vegetables. Instead of pizza, pasta and sandwiches, think meat-and-veggie-based stir-fries, sautés, soups and salads.

- **Include fruits, nuts and seeds in your diet.** Fresh and unsweetened frozen fruits are part of the Paleolithic diet, but avoid the more processed types – canned fruits and fruit juices

– and minimize or avoid dried fruits. You can also use nuts and seeds as snacks or ingredients in dishes, but avoid peanuts, which actually are legumes.

• **Don't eat dairy foods or sweeteners.** In place of cow's milk or cream, try unsweetened coconut milk or homemade almond milk. In place of butter, use coconut butter or olive oil. Keep sugar, other refined sweeteners, and artificial sweeteners out of your diet, including hidden sources of sweeteners, such as sweetened drinks.

• **Try nut-flour baked goods.** Pancakes, muffins and crackers can be made with almond flour, hazelnut flour and/or coconut flour, with other helpful ingredients such as eggs, coconut butter, and fruit. For some people such as Cindy, these additional modifications take the gluten-free diet to a new level in providing therapeutic benefit.

The nutritional profile of grass-fed meats more closely approximates the nutritional profile of the game meats that were in the Paleolithic or Stone Age hunter-gatherer diet. Grass-fed meats have less total fat than grain-fed meats, so it's important not to overcook them. Here is an easy recipe to try using grass-fed ground lamb.

Serve meatballs with steamed or roasted asparagus spears or on top of steamed or lightly sautéed spinach and garlic in olive oil, and drizzle meatball au jus on top of both. You can also slice leftover meatballs, reheat them, and add them on top of a large salad with red onion, cucumber, tomato, and romaine lettuce with lemon juice, olive oil and herb dressing.

Grass-Fed Lamb Meatballs Florentine

1 lb. organic grass-fed ground lamb
3 garlic cloves, smashed and minced
1/3 cup fresh baby spinach leaves, chopped
1/4 cup fresh parsley leaves, minced
1/4 cup fresh basil leaves, minced
Unrefined sea salt or Herbamare herb seasoning
   salt to taste

Preheat oven to 350 degrees. In a bowl, knead together the lamb, garlic, spinach, parsley and basil until they are well mixed. Form into 1-inch meatballs, tucking in any herb or spinach pieces that are sticking out into the ground meat. Arrange in even rows in an 8" x 11-1/2" x 2" baking dish. Bake on a medium rack for 18 to 20 minutes or until done to your liking. Sprinkle with salt to taste. Makes 24 balls. Serves 4.

Chapter 24 – December:

The Gift of Gluten Free

Checking your holiday gift list and need ideas for people on your list who eat gluten free? Don't worry, there are numerous choices to fit many different tastes at your local natural foods store. When you play Santa, look for safe gluten-free gifts like these:

• **Teas to warm the soul.** For welcome gifts for the cool winter season, choose single-ingredient teas, such as green tea or chamomile tea, or herbal tea combinations that are labeled gluten-free, such as Good Earth Caffeine-Free Sweet and Spicy – with or without a coffee mug. For extra Christmas spirit, give a box of holiday tea, such as Celestial Seasonings peppermint-flavored Candy Cane Lane Tea.

• **A basket of fruit to refresh the body.** Have an arrangement made up or make your own with an inexpensive basket and assorted seasonal fruit, such as oranges, pears, apples, bananas and kiwi. A bag of dried cranberries can add a nice seasonal touch.

• **Nuts to satisfy the appetite.** Nuts, such as organic shelled pecans, are a great snack, appetizer, or ingredient to use in recipes, which makes them a nice present, too. Want extra holiday flair? Buy a few nutcrackers and assorted unshelled nuts – a great gift to give to someone who will have guests or family coming for the holidays.

• **A special dessert to make a get-together sweeter.** People who eat gluten free have to skip common desserts so often that they really appreciate getting desserts that they know are safe for them to eat. For an extra-nice surprise, consider buying a friend or family member who eats gluten free a dessert appropriate for the season, such as Fabe's Gluten-Free Vegan Apple Pie or Pamela's Products Ginger Cookies or Butter Shortbread. Or make your own dessert for them, such as your favorite homemade gluten-free pie, cookies, or cake.

• **A gluten-free book to educate the mind.** A gluten-free diet book or cookbook is a thoughtful gift, especially for a friend who has just begun a gluten-free diet and seems overwhelmed. To get that person off to a healthy start, consider making a gluten-free care basket with a book and a few gluten-free baking supplies or gluten-free snacks.

• **Bath care products to pamper the body.** If you'd like to steer clear of food-related gifts, try health and beauty products. Good choices tolerated by even most allergic people are luxurious essential-oil-based bath oils, such as Aura Cacia Comforting Vanilla Aromatherapy Massage Body Oil, or relaxing bath salts, such as Batherapy Lavender Bath Salts.

• **Stocking stuffers for fun.** A gluten-free chocolate bar, such as Enjoy Life Foods' boom-Choco-Boom bar or refined-sugar-free Cherry Chocolate Bumble Bar, makes a sweet stocking stuffer. Or try a small festive personal care product, such as Loofah-Art's colorful bath scrubbies or Kiss My Face Holiday Lip Balm Duo Pack (in Vanilla Sugar and Cranberry Spice).

• **Organic cotton clothes that help the environment.** Made with cotton not sprayed with all the pesticides found in commercial cotton, an organic cotton shirt or bathrobe is a present that virtually everyone feels good getting because it is better for us and for the planet.

• **A gift certificate from a natural foods store.** If you're unsure about what to buy, a gift certificate is always a good choice. It's a gift that many people appreciate the most because they can use it on anything they want – from grass-fed meat, to gluten-free crackers, to kosher foods, to shower gels they can pick out themselves.

Want to share something rich and decadent for the holidays? Create unique chocolate balls by combining cocoa powder, nut butter and dried fruit. They require a bit of patience to make but they look wonderful on a serving plate, especially surrounded by fresh strawberries and raspberries. They are also rich, so you don't need many.

No-Bake Dried Fruit-Cocoa Balls

1/2 cup pitted sulfite-free prunes
4 Tbsp. dried unsweetened Bing cherries
3 Tbsp. unsweetened cocoa powder
3 Tbsp. roasted almond butter, creamy style
3 tsp. Frontier Herbs Alcohol-Free Vanilla Flavor
1/4 to 1/2 tsp. ground cinnamon
2 Tbsp. chopped pecans (optional)
1/2 cup finely grated unsweetened, sulfite-free
    organic coconut

Cut prunes in quarters and dried cherries in halves. Mix 1 Tbsp. of the cocoa powder in with the dried fruit (to keep it from sticking together as much) and chop the mixture until minced. Slide the chopped mixture into a mixing bowl; add remaining cocoa, almond butter, vanilla flavor, and cinnamon; and mix. Put on disposable plastic gloves for easier handling, if desired, and knead the mixture until well combined, adding in the pecans at the end. Roll the mixture into one-inch balls and coat each ball in coconut. Refrigerate overnight or for at least an hour to set, but bring chocolate balls to room temperature for an hour or two before serving for best flavor. Makes 12 balls. Recipe can be doubled.

Note: If you have a food processor, you can use it to make this dessert easier. Drop the prunes and dried cherries through the feed hole one by one, scrape the processor bowl, and add remaining ingredients except for the pecans and coconut.

Appendix A:

Straight Talk on Testing for Gluten Sensitivity and Carbohydrate Sensitivity

Testing for Gluten Sensitivity

Let's be honest: Trying to get diagnosed with gluten sensitivity through traditional means is an exercise in frustration. To begin with, the average doctor denies that the condition even exists. If you prod your doctor, he may order a blood test to screen for antibodies involved in celiac disease, the gluten-related autoimmune disease. The antibody tests done are those that test for a reaction to gluten (IgA and IgG gliadin antibodies) and those that test for tissue damage (IgA tissue transglutaminase and/or endomysial antibodies). If all these tests come back positive, your doctor will refer you to a gastroenterologist for an intestinal biopsy for "official" confirmation of celiac disease. (However, as one doctor told me, there may be some financial motivation to keep such a highly paid procedure as the gold standard of diagnosis.)

If the tests for tissue damage come back negative, your doctor will tell you that you don't have celiac disease and will typically ignore the results of the other tests, even if they are positive. However, if either of the gliadin antibody tests is positive, you *are* gluten sensitive (also called gluten intolerant), but most people simply aren't told this.

But take note: *Even if you test negative on the IgG and IgA gliadin antibody tests, you still could be gluten intolerant.* That's because you could have a different type of reaction, an allergy to gluten. To test for all the types of reactions gluten may cause, a few doctors who specialize in gluten intolerance use laboratories that test IgA, IgG, and IgE antibody levels in the blood to not just gliadin (a part of gluten) but also to wheat and the other gluten grains. But many people can't find a doctor who will be open to ordering this spectrum of antibody tests, so the tests are out of the question for most people.

If you test negative on IgA and IgG gliadin tests and would like further testing – or if you want to try to get a diagnosis of gluten sensitivity without going through the process most people go through that I just described – you might want to order a gluten sensitivity stool test from Enterolab.com. The test kit will be mailed to you, and you can give your sample in the privacy of your own home and mail it back to the company to get the results. There are few studies on the gluten sensitivity stool test, and it is not acknowledged or accepted by most doctors. However, the test was developed by a medical doctor who saw the need for a different type of test for the many people who did not have celiac disease but still reacted to gluten. I wrote about the Enterolab gluten sensitivity stool test in *Going Against the Grain*, and many readers and clients who didn't get answers any other way have been greatly helped by ordering this test. The stool test seems to pick up cases of gluten sensitivity earlier in the disease process than blood tests.

Research is continuing into gluten sensitivity and how to test for the condition, and new tests may be coming. But the best test of all may be whether you respond positively to a healthy gluten-free diet. (Of course, if you do a gluten-free diet trial and eat junky refined gluten-free foods and still feel badly, that is no real surprise and certainly not a fair test of whether the gluten-free diet is therapeutic for you.) If you take gluten out of your diet the right way, and find that uncomfortable, perplexing or longstanding symptoms go away, that really should be all the proof you need that you have gluten intolerance and that a gluten-free diet is therapeutic for you. The merits of a gluten-free diet trial is that it's not expensive, you don't have to fight with your doctor to do it, and most notably, you get to see firsthand how much better you feel when you eat gluten free. That usually makes people believers in the power of gluten-free eating far better than any lab test results can. I know it definitely did for me.

Other health practitioners who specialize in gluten intolerance are coming to the same conclusion that patients should see if symptoms respond to a gluten-free diet. Dr. Rodney Ford, a specialist in gluten illness from New Zealand, says we shouldn't be focused on the gut tissue tests. The criteria used to diagnose celiac disease – in other words, the presence of small intestine damage and of tissue damage antibodies in the blood – does not matter in terms of predicting who would be helped by the gluten-free diet, according to Dr. Ford. We should be focused on treating the symptoms that develop when gluten-sensitive people eat gluten and that go away when people stop eating gluten. The symptoms of celiac disease and gluten sensitivity are the same. The only difference is that celiac disease has been shown to involve gut damage.

The one big drawback of a gluten-free diet experiment is you might not see that the gluten-free diet is therapeutic for you if you happen to have silent celiac disease – a condition in which there is damage to the gut but without any or many noticeable symptoms. If you have a condition that is a common complication of celiac disease, such as iron-deficiency anemia, osteoporosis, infertility, or an autoimmune disease, be sure to get the blood tests to screen for celiac disease first before eliminating gluten from your diet to rule out silent celiac disease.

Testing for Carbohydrate Sensitivity

Many people who are gluten sensitive are carbohydrate sensitive, too, but don't know it. Trying to get diagnosed with a blood-sugar- or insulin-related condition such as prediabetes is relatively easy and certainly easier than it used to be. But most people, including many doctors, don't know the beginning signs of the carbohydrate sensitivity disease process, which is why carbohydrate sensitivity in the earlier stages is often missed.

Fortunately, the easiest way to determine carbohydrate sensitivity is through your symptoms. By paying attention to your symptoms and also to heart-disease risk factors that are indicated on standard blood test results, you can connect the dots to determine that you are carbohydrate sensitive to one degree or another, even if your doctor doesn't.

Doctors who specialize in insulin-related health conditions sometimes test fasting and two-hour post-meal levels of insulin and perform other specialized tests to get more specifics on the degree of insulin resistance that patients have. These tests can be helpful but aren't necessary as symptoms are the main indicators.

The following are some common signs and symptoms of carbohydrate sensitivity, starting at the beginning of the list with earlier indicators and continuing to more advanced signs. The more of these you have, especially symptoms toward the bottom of the list, the more carbohydrate sensitive you likely are.

Common Signs and Symptoms of Carbohydrate Sensitivity

Cravings for sweets or grains, including gluten-free
   whole grains
Difficulty stopping to eat sweets or grains once you start
Sleepiness an hour or two after meals
Lack of mental focus in between meals
Mood swings, irritability, or a shaky feeling
   in between meals
Erratic swings in energy
Overweight, especially through the waistline
High blood triglyceride levels (above 100 mg/dL)
Low HDL cholesterol levels

Poor triglyceride-to-HDL cholesterol ratios (above 2)

High blood pressure (consistently above 140/90)

Elevated blood sugar levels (fasting glucose above
  100 mg/dL)

A diagnosis of metabolic syndrome

A diagnosis of prediabetes or type 2 diabetes

A diagnosis of polycystic ovary syndrome (PCOS)

Just as gluten sensitivity and the symptoms and conditions associated with it clear up on a gluten-free diet, carbohydrate sensitivity and the symptoms and conditions associated with it gradually clear up on a grain-free, sugar-free diet, especially the Paleolithic hunter-gatherer diet. (See Chapter 23 for more details.) If you need more evidence that you are carbohydrate sensitive, just try avoiding all sugars and even gluten-free grains, and eating mostly poultry, fish, meat and vegetables for two weeks. See if some of your symptoms start to improve or go away. If they do, you have tested yourself and have gotten the answer that you are likely carbohydrate sensitive and that a grain-free, sugar-free diet is therapeutic for you.

People are sometimes scared to try these diet trials on their own without their doctor's approval. They mistakenly think cutting out grains could somehow be harmful to them. But the original diet of man was free of grains and that is what the human body evolved on. So, there is no harm in testing yourself and seeing what happens. The results of this test might pleasantly surprise and amaze you.

Appendix B:

Substitutions for Common Wheat-Based Foods

Pasta

Gluten free: Brown rice pasta (such as Lundberg Farms, Tinkyada and others)

Gluten free and more nutritious: Brown rice pasta with flaxseed (such as Hodgson Mill)

Grain free and low carb: Spaghetti squash (see Chapter 5 for more info); Vegetable "Spaghetti" recipe in Chapter 5; Sea Tangle Kelp Noodles.

Bread

Gluten free: Bread made primarily with whole-grain rice or other gluten-free grains (such as Food for Life Forbidden Rice Bread, Bhutanese Red Rice Bread, and Rice-Almond Bread)

Grain free and low carb: Homemade bread made with eggs and nut flour or coconut flour.

Tortillas

Gluten free: Brown rice tortillas; organic, non-GMO yellow corn or blue corn tortillas.

Grain free and low carb: Raw Makery Rawtillas (made with sprouted brown and golden flax seeds, sunflower seeds and sesame seeds).

Crackers/Chips

Gluten free: Mary's Gone Crackers gluten-free crackers and Sticks & Twigs; Crunchmaster Original Multi-Seed Crackers; Blue Diamond Nut Thins; organic, non-GMO yellow corn or blue corn tortilla chips.

Gluten free and more nutritious: Raw Makery Stix, Krispys and Bread (made with sprouted buckwheat and seeds); organic, non-GMO corn tortilla chips with flaxseed.

Gluten free and certified low glycemic: Beanitos Black Bean Chips and Pinto Bean & Flax Chips, which are both corn free.

Grain free and low carb: Raw vegetable sticks, such as carrot sticks, celery sticks, and cucumber rounds; homemade crackers made out of nut flour (see recipes for Savory Pecan Flatbread Rounds and Egg-Free Caraway Nut Crackers in Chapter 21);

flaxseed crackers such as Foods Alive Flax Crackers and Go Raw Flax Snax; and Kaia Foods Kale Chips in several varieties, including Sea Salt & Vinegar and Chili Lime.

Appendix C:

Resources

Recommended Books for More Information

Going Against the Grain: How Reducing and Avoiding Grains Can Revitalize Your Health by Melissa Diane Smith

Syndrome X: The Complete Nutritional Program to Prevent and Reverse Insulin Resistance by Jack Challem, Burton Berkson, and Melissa Diane Smith

User's Guide to Preventing and Reversing Diabetes Naturally by Melissa Diane Smith

The Gluten Syndrome: Is Wheat Causing You Harm? by Dr. Rodney Ford

Healthier Without Wheat: A New Understanding of Wheat Allergies, Celiac Disease, and Non-Celiac Gluten Intolerance by Dr. Stephen Wangen

The Paleo Diet by Loren Cordain, Ph.D.

Cooking with Coconut Flour by Bruce Fife, N.D.

The Grain-Free Gourmet by Jodi Bager and Jenny Lass

Recommended DVDs for More Information

Food, Inc. (2008 documentary motion picture) by Robert Kenner (director) and Robert Kenner and Elise Pearlstein (writers)

King Corn (2007 documentary motion picture) by Aaron Wolf (director) and Curt Ellis and Ian Cheney (writers)

Recommended Websites for More Information

www.AgainstTheGrainNutrition.com

Melissa's website to spread the word about the healing power of Against the Grain Nutrition. It houses her private online Going Against the Grain Group that contains a searchable database of helpful articles for ongoing support and her open-to-the-public blog and free every-other-month newsletter, *Nutrition News & Notes*, which provides summaries of recent against-the-grain research, items in the news, and occasional opinion pieces. You can use the search engine on the blog to look for up-to-date and in-depth articles on topics covered in this book, including gluten sensitivity, celiac disease, insulin resistance, overweight, type 2 diabetes, the hazards of genetically modified corn, and the benefits of gluten-free and grain-free diets.

www.MelissaDianeSmith.com

Melissa's original website with information on her background, books, speaking services, and nutrition services that are available to people across the country over the phone. This is the site to contact Melissa if you're interested in her long-distance nutrition consultations or coaching programs, or for public speaking inquiries, interviews by the media, or consulting for food product development. Also, if you would like your success story shared with visitors to this site, please summarize your story in a few paragraphs and send it to info@melissadianesmith.com.

www.Celiac.com

A helpful site with wide-ranging informative articles on the gluten-free lifestyle, with a Safe Gluten-Free Food List and Unsafe Foods and Ingredients List that are kept up to date and are good to bookmark or print out for handy reference.

Also on this site at *www.celiac.com/categories/Journal-of-Gluten-Sensitivity/*, you can learn about the *Journal of Gluten*

Sensitivity edited by Dr. Ron Hoggan. The journal is a quarterly research-oriented publication for those with celiac disease or gluten sensitivity that is available by subscription.

www.CenterForFoodAllergies.com

A website that gives good information on food allergies and food allergy testing by gluten and food allergy specialist Stephen Wangen, N.D.

www.DoctorGluten.com

Gluten sensitivity specialist Dr. Rodney Ford's website with information on his Food Allergy eClinic, a place to get expert individual food allergy help and blood test result interpretation online, and on the Doctor Gluten Project, which was created to help spread the word about the harmful effects of gluten.

www.EnteroLab.com

A site to order a conduct-at-home stool test for gluten sensitivity, celiac disease, malabsorption, and more.

www.Gluten.net

The Gluten Intolerance Group of North America, also known as GIG, provides support to people with any type of gluten intolerance, including celiac disease, dermatitis herpetiformis, and other gluten sensitivities. It puts out a quarterly newsletter and is best known for its Gluten-Free Certification Organization (GFCO.org), which certifies gluten-free companies and products based on strict criteria and on-site inspections, and for the Gluten-Free Restaurant Awareness Program (Glutenfreerestaurants.org), which has developed strict criteria for accrediting restaurants for their gluten-free awareness and service.

www.NonGMOShoppingGuide.com

A consumer-oriented site co-produced by The Institute for Responsible Technology and The Center for Food Safety. It has helpful information on why we should avoid genetically modified foods (including corn), how to avoid them, and a free Non-GMO shopping guide you can download.

Other Helpful Celiac-Specific Organizations

www.CeliacCenter.org
The University of Maryland Center for Celiac Research, which is led by leading researcher Alessio Fasano, M.D.

www.Celiac.org
The Celiac Disease Foundation

www.CSAceliacs.org
Celiac Sprue Association

www.Celiac.ca
Canadian Celiac Association

www.SouthernArizonaCeliacSupport.org
Southern Arizona Celiac Support, a particularly active chapter of the Celiac Sprue Association

www.TriumphDining.com
Triumph Dining

The site where you can order Triumph Dining cards in ten different languages and *The Essential Gluten-Free Restaurant Guide*, two good resources for dining safely in restaurants in your hometown or when you're traveling.

Against-the-Grain Foods

You should be able to find or special-order most if not all of the gluten-free and grain-free products mentioned in this book in a natural food store in your area.

The simpler and more natural and nutritious the foods in food products, the better they are for us. The following companies offer foods that are in keeping with that philosophy and deserve special mention for the nutritious, innovative, minimally processed whole-food products they offer. Many people who feel best on a reduced-carbohydrate or grain-free diet find it worth placing online orders from the companies below if they have trouble getting some of the foods that these companies offer.

Kaia Foods

www.KaiaFoods.com

A company that uses minimally processed organic ingredients to create extremely nutritious snack foods, such as Sprouted Sunflower Seeds and vitamin A-packed Kale Chips in four tasty flavors. (What a great way to get more vegetables in the diet!) My clients love the taste of these foods and feel great after eating them because of the power-packed nutrition they provide.

Nutiva

www.Nutiva.com

This company sells organic chia seeds and hemp seeds and makes what is largely considered the best-tasting and best-selling organic extra virgin coconut oil and a new, "melt in your mouth" whole-food product from organic whole coconut called Coconut Manna. The delicious new food contains 16% fiber, 7% protein and nourishing fats, and can be eaten a spoonful at a time as a low-carb treat or used to make up dreamy, non-dairy "creamy," sugar-free or minimally sweetened desserts.

Raw Makery
www.RawMakery.com

A company that makes a newly developed, tasty, bendable and particularly innovative Rawtilla made out of sprouted brown and golden flax seeds, sunflower seeds and sesame seeds. This tortilla substitute is rich in fiber and omega-3 fatty acids and low in carbs.

Sea Tangle Kelp Noodles
www.KelpNoodles.com

A very versatile, ready-to-eat, ultra-low-carb food that is rich in nutrients, including iodine, which is needed for healthy thyroid function. The noodles are made out of kelp but have a completely neutral taste and are exceptionally easy to use. They are a godsend for people who want pasta without the grains or carbs normally present in pasta.

Numerous gluten-free products, such as the following, can usually be purchased through Amazon.com:

Beanitos Black Bean Chips
Bob's Red Mill Coconut Flour
Featherweight Baking Powder
Foods Alive flax crackers, such as Maple & Cinnamon, Italian Zest, or Mexican varieties
Frontier Herbs Alcohol-Free Vanilla Flavor
Go Raw Bars, Flax Snax, Sprouted Sunflower Seeds & Pumpkin Seeds, and Super Cookies
Kaia Foods Sprouted Sunflower Seeds
Mary's Gone Crackers and Sticks & Twigs
NOW Foods Almond Flour
Olade stevia-sweetened beverage
Organic coconut oil, such as Nutiva or Nature's Way EFA-Gold
Pure Food Bar
Raw Makery Krispys, Biskits, Stix, Bread and Cookies
ReBar Original Fruit & Vegetable Bar

Appendix D:

Putting It All Together: Sample Menus

Here are examples of different types of meals you can have according to the seasons and different circumstances that may be going on in your life.

A Winter Weekend Day
(when you're relaxing and hanging around the house)

Brunch

Homemade turkey sausage patties with ground fennel and sage
Almond Pancakes (recipe in Chapter 1) with sliced pear

Snack

A bowl of vegetable or chicken soup
or
Celery sticks with almond butter

Dinner

Organic pot roast with carrots, celery, onions, red potato and green beans made in vegetable juice

---

A Spring Day
(when you're eating lighter and trying to shed unwanted pounds)

Breakfast

Savory Quinoa Hash (recipe in Chapter 1) with diced turkey breast meat
A small bowl of fresh strawberries and blueberries

Lunch

Herbes de Provence Chicken Strips (recipe in Chapter 20) or Grass-Fed Lamb Meatballs Florentine (recipe in Chapter 23)
Steamed Globe artichoke with lemon juice-olive oil dressing or a vinaigrette
Roasted asparagus spears with olive oil

Snack

Sprouted sunflower seeds

Dinner

Filet of Sole Florentine (recipe in Chapter 3)
A side salad with mixed baby greens, sliced cucumber, red
onion and radish and lemon juice-olive oil dressing

A Summer Day
(when the weather is hot and you're short on time)

Breakfast

A hard-boiled omega-3-enriched egg or leftover slices of
chicken sprinkled with unrefined sea salt
Melissa's Quick High-Fiber Muesli (recipe in Chapter 17) made
with chopped nectarine
Or
Celery sticks with almond butter

Lunch

Chicken and Strawberry Salad with Cilantro-Lime Dressing
(recipe in Chapter 19)
Or
A gluten-free turkey sandwich on a Raw Makery Dill or Onion
Rawtilla (tortilla substitute) with lettuce and mustard, assorted
fresh vegetable sticks, and Kaia Foods Kale Chips

Snack

Macadamia nuts or pecans

Dinner

Cool Noodle Tabouli for One with shrimp added (recipe in
Chapter 6 – increase the amount if not eating by yourself)
Carrot sticks and cucumber rounds

An Autumn Day
(when you feel like cooking more)

Breakfast

Leftover chicken stir-fry with assorted Chinese vegetables and brown rice

Lunch

Baked sea bass with olive oil and dill
Green beans with toasted almonds

Dinner

Pork roast with sage
Butternut Squash with Fresh Sage (recipe in Chapter 11)
Steamed Broccoli and Cauliflower

The following are examples of meals for various seasonal occasions and major holidays.

A Football or Other Sporting Event Party

Broiled turkey and grass-fed hamburgers on lettuce topped with either sautéed garlic mushrooms or with sliced red onion and tomato and homemade guacamole
Beanitos Pinto Bean & Flax Chips with guacamole and salsa
Carrot strips
Bowl of roasted almonds and macadamia nuts
Bowl of small apples

Easter meal

Roast spring chicken or roast leg of lamb with herbs
Pink Rice Pilaf with Roasted Asparagus and Mushrooms (recipe in Chapter 16)
Or
Greek Spinach and Rice (recipe in Chapter 10)
Peas and carrots
Greek salad with or without the feta cheese

Memorial Day or July 4th Picnic

Herbes de Provence Chicken Strips (recipe in Chapter 20)
Greek Potato Salad (recipe in Chapter 18)
Or
Cool Noodle Tabouli (recipe in Chapter 6 – increase the
amount for the picnic)
Carrot and celery sticks
Fresh Bing cherries or watermelon cubes
Olade beverage or sparkling mineral water

A simple Thanksgiving feast

Roast turkey with natural au jus or gravy made with arrowroot
Chestnut Stuffing or Savory Stuffing (recipes in Chapter 12) or
Baked yams or sweet potatoes drizzled with macadamia nut oil,
Spectrum Organics Roasted Hazelnut Oil, or butter, and
ground cinnamon
Fruit-juice-concentrate-sweetened cranberry sauce
Steamed broccoli
Pecan-Pear Autumn Sundaes (recipe in Chapter 11)

Christmas Day meal

A salad with green leaf lettuce, toasted hazelnuts and chopped apple
Garlic-Rosemary Pork Roast
Pink Rice Pilaf with Roasted Asparagus and Mushrooms (recipe in Chapter 16)
Or
Savory Stuffing (recipe in Chapter 12)
Green beans
Pumpkin pie with a gluten-free crust or, the easier alternative, with no crust

New Year's Eve party food

Chicken and beef kabobs with red onion, red pepper and mushrooms with hummus or Trader Joe's Tahini Sauce for dipping
Cauliflower with Lemon-Tahini Sauce (recipe in Chapter 22)
Sautéed mushrooms with garlic in olive oil
Olives
Kaia Foods Kale Chips
Party platter with orange and apple wedges and pieces of Pecan Pie and Cinnamon Roll Larabars

Selected References

Bernardo D, Garrote JA, Fernandez-Salazar L, et al. Is gliadin really safe for non-coeliac individuals? Production of interleukin 15 in biopsy culture from non-coeliac individuals with gliadin peptides. *Gut*, 2007;56:889-890.

Challem J, Berkson B, Smith MD. *Syndrome X: The Complete Nutritional Program to Prevent and Reverse Insulin Resistance.* New York: John Wiley & Sons, 2000.

Cordain, L. The nutritional characteristics of a contemporary diet based upon Paleolithic food groups. *Journal of the American Nutraceutical Association*, 2002; 5:15-24.

Dickey W, Kearney N. Overweight in celiac disease: prevalence, clinical characteristics, and effect of a gluten-free diet. *American Journal of Gastroenterology*, 2006; 101:2365-9.

Ford, Rodney. *The Gluten Syndrome: Is Wheat Causing You Harm?* Christchurch, New Zealand: RRS Global Ltd., 2007.

Ford RPK. The gluten syndrome: A neurological disease. *Medical Hypothesis* (2009), doi:10.1016/j.mehy.2009.03.037.

Ford, Rodney K. Which serological tests best identify gluten reactions? *Journal of Pediatric Gastroenterology & Nutrition*, 2009;Vol. 49, suppl 1, p. E14.

Frassetto LA, Schloetter M, Mietus-Synder M, et al. Metabolic and physiologic improvements from consuming a Paleolithic, hunter-gatherer type diet. *European Journal of Clinical Nutrition* advance online publication, 11 February 2009;doi:10.1038/ejcn.2009.4.

Jonsson, T, Granfeldt Y, Ahren B, et al. Beneficial effects of a Paleolithic diet on cardiovascular risk factors in type 2 diabetes: A randomized cross-over pilot study. *Cardiovascular Diabetology*, 2009 July 16; 8: 35 doi:10.1186/1475-2840-8-35.

Kenner, Robert (director) & Kenner, Robert, & Pearlstein, Elise (writers). *Food, Inc.* [documentary motion picture]. USA: Docudrama, 2008.

Lindeberg S, Jonsson T, Granfeldt Y, et al. A Paleolithic diet improves glucose intolerance more than a Mediterranean-like diet in individuals with ischemic heart disease. *Diabetologia*, 2007;50:1795-1807.

Personal communications with Rodney Ford, M.D., November 6-10, 2009, in Tucson, AZ.

Personal email communication with Kenneth Fine, M.D., January 6, 2010.

Personal phone interview with Alessio Fasano, M.D., January 13, 2010.

Personal phone interview with Steve Wangen, N.D., January 14, 2010.

Rampertab SD, Pooran N, Brar P, et al. Trends in the presentation of celiac disease. *American Journal of Medicine,* 2006;119;355.e9-355.e14.

Roe, Sam. Children at risk in food roulette. Mislabeling, lax oversight threaten people with allergies. *Chicago Tribune,* November 21, 2008.

Sapone A, Lammers K, Casolaro V, et al. Gluten sensitivity is associated to activation of the innate but not Th1/Th17 immune response to gluten exposure. *Journal of Pediatric Gastroenterology & Nutrition,* 2009;Vol. 49, suppl 1, p. E14.

Smith, Melissa Diane. *Going Against the Grain.* New York: McGraw-Hill/Contemporary Books, 2002.

Spiroux de Vendomois J, Roulliet F, Cellier D, Seralini GE. A Comparison of the Effects of Three GM Corn Varieties on Mammalian Health. *International Journal of Biological Sciences,* 2009;5(7):706-726.

Telega GT, Bennet TR, Werlin S. Emerging clinical patterns in the presentation of celiac disease. *Archives of Pediatric and Adolescent Medicine,* 2008;162:164-168.

Wangen, Stephen. *Healthier Without Wheat: A New Understanding of Wheat Allergies, Celiac Disease, and Non-Celiac Gluten Intolerance.* Seattle, Washington: Innate Health Publishing, 2009.

Woolf, Aaron (director) & Ellis, Curt, and Cheney, Ian (writers). *King Corn* [documentary motion picture]. USA: Docudrama, 2007.

Recipe Index

About the Author

Melissa Diane Smith is an internationally known nutritionist who specializes in grain-related conditions, including gluten sensitivity, celiac disease, other autoimmune diseases, and grain allergies and addictions, and sugar-related health conditions, including excess weight, metabolic syndrome, polycystic ovary syndrome, diabetes and prediabetes. Her philosophy is that food is our best medicine and she counsels clients long distance over the phone and gives presentations to healthcare professional and mainstream audiences throughout the United States and Canada. She also counsels clients in person in Tucson, Arizona, writes an *Against the Grain Nutrition News & Notes* newsletter, and hosts an online Going Against The Grain Group database of articles with news and food-oriented support for people who eat against the grain.

Melissa is the author of the groundbreaking *Going Against the Grain: How Reducing and Avoiding Grains Can Revitalize Your Health*. She also is the author of *User's Guide to Preventing and Reversing Diabetes Naturally* and the coauthor of *Syndrome X: The Complete Nutritional Program to Prevent and Reverse Insulin Resistance.*

Melissa has written nutrition-related articles for numerous magazines and publications, and has been the Go Gluten Free columnist for *Better Nutrition* magazine for more than two years. Her work has been written about in *The Los Angeles Times, Chicago Tribune, Woman's World, First for Women* magazine, *New Zealand Woman's Weekly*, and on *WebMD*. She also has spoken at numerous conferences, including the American Academy of Physician Assistants annual conference, the "Polycystic Ovary Syndrome: The Perfect Endocrine Storm" conference, Natural Products Expo West, the Nutritional Pathways to Health and Healing Conference for First Nations People in Edmonton, Canada, and the Australasian Integrative Medicine Association conference in Auckland, New Zealand.

Melissa combines the investigative research skills she honed in journalism school with her nutrition training and more than fifteen years of clinical nutrition experience to stay up to date on cutting-edge nutrition research and to provide clients with nutrition advice that is based on recent research and personalized for their needs and health goals.

Organizations with public speaking or special event book signing inquiries and media members that are interested in conducting interviews with Melissa should write to speaking@melissadianesmith.com. To inquire about Melissa's services for consulting for food product development, write to info@melissadianesmith.com. If you're interested in personalized nutrition consultations or coaching programs over the phone with Melissa, view the rates for her nutrition services on her website, and if you'd like to get started working with her, write to mds@melissadianesmith.com.

CPSIA information can be obtained
at www.ICGtesting.com
Printed in the USA
BVHW041100080721
611461BV00005B/121